Syndrome X

Other books by Jack Challem

The Natural Health Guide to Beating the Supergerms
All About Vitamins
All About Vitamin E
All About Carotenoids

Other books by Burton Berkson, M.D., Ph.D.

The Alpha Lipoic Acid Breakthrough
All About B Vitamins

Other books by Melissa Diane Smith

Why Am I Always So Tired?
All About Zinc
All About Vitamin E

Syndrome X

The Complete Nutritional Program to Prevent and Reverse Insulin Resistance

Jack Challem
Burton Berkson, M.D., Ph.D.
Melissa Diane Smith

John Wiley & Sons, Inc.
New York • Chichester • Weinheim • Brisbane • Singapore • Toronto

Published by John Wiley & Sons, Inc.
Published simultaneously in Canada

The Anti-X™ Diet and the Anti-X Extra-Healing™ Diet are trademarks of Jack Challem, Burton Berkson, and Melissa Diane Smith. The Nutrition Reporter™ is a trademark of Jack Challem.

This publication is designed to provide accurate and authoritative information in regard to the subject matter covered. It is sold with the understanding that the publisher is not engaged in rendering professional services. If professional advice or other expert assistance is required, the services of a competent professional should be sought.

Library of Congress Cataloging-in-Publication Data:

Challem, Jack.
    Syndrome X: the complete nutritional program to prevent and reverse
  insulin resistance / Jack Challem, Burton Berkson, Melissa Diane Smith.
      p. cm.
  Includes index.
  ISBN 0-471-35835-5 (cloth : alk. paper)
  ISBN 0-471-39858-6 (paper)
    1. Insulin resistance—Diet therapy. 2. Insulin resistance—Complications—
  Prevention. I. Berkson, Burton. II. Smith, Melissa Diane. III. Title.
  RC662.4.C47   2000
  616.3'998—dc21   99-049639

Printed in the United States of America

15 14 13 12

CONTENTS

PREFACE

IF YOU HAVE never heard of Syndrome X, you're probably wondering, What is this mysterious condition, and why should I be concerned about it?

The answer is very simple: You may already be suffering from it.

We believe that Syndrome X is a disorder most people seriously risk developing by the time they reach middle age, if not before. Syndrome X can explain why you feel lousy today—such as being tired and fuzzy-minded. It can also age you faster than normal, setting the stage for catastrophic health problems, such as heart disease, diabetes, Alzheimer's disease, cancer, and other age-related diseases.

A *syndrome* is a condition defined by a cluster of related symptoms or disorders. In this case, Syndrome X refers specifically to a group of health problems that includes *insulin resistance* (the inability to properly deal with dietary carbohydrates such as sugars), as well as one or more other problems, such as abnormal blood fats (elevated cholesterol or triglycerides), overweight, and high blood pressure.

For years, doctors have known that each of these health problems can increase the risk of other diseases, such as heart disease and diabetes. Until relatively recently, however, they failed to connect the dots and see these health problems as part of a syndrome. We now know that eating large amounts of dietary carbohydrates (such as sweets, pastas, and breads) can raise cholesterol, triglyceride, and insulin levels. We know also that elevated insulin can promote obesity and high blood pressure. Because these problems are related and tend to occur in clusters, they form a syndrome.

X, of course, has always represented the unknown, whether it referred to hidden conspiracies in the *X-Files* television show or the unknown integer in algebra. Researchers named the syndrome "X" when it was first recognized, but still largely unproved and mysterious. Today, Syndrome X is no longer a mystery. It is a frightfully common, and often ignored, disorder that can derail your health.

The good news is that it does not have to harm you. Syndrome X is primarily a nutritional disease caused by eating the wrong types of foods. You have the power to modify your lifestyle to protect yourself against Syndrome X, and this book will tell you how you can do so relatively easily.

If you're tired of being overweight; having high triglycerides, high cholesterol, or high blood pressure; feeling lousy after meals; and seeing your health spin out of control—and not knowing why—it's time for you to delve into this book. The program we've put together involves diet, light physical activity, and the use of supplements. We call it, quite simply, the Anti-X program. We know it works because it has worked for *us*—helping us to shed unwanted pounds, get our blood sugar under control, and feel more energized. Since the first edition of this book was published in January 2000, we have also heard many wonderful success stories from readers. One of the most powerful and touching responses began with "Thank you for saving my life. I was slowly dying until I found your book . . . "

Such dramatic turnarounds are especially poignant given the disastrous state of modern nutrition and health. In August 2000, a leading medical journal reported that the incidence of adult-onset diabetes, one of the major consequences of Syndrome X, increased by a previously unheard-of 33 percent in the United States over the last decade—and by a mind-boggling 70 percent among people in their 30s!

With all the current headlines and fanfare about gene research, and the smoke and mirrors of pharmaceutical advertising, we must remember that diabetes and Syndrome X can be rectified simply by eating healthier foods. Other low-carbohydrate diet programs touch on these issues, but none of them tackles insulin resistance and Syndrome X in such a balanced and comprehensive way as our program does. The Anti-X program addresses Syndrome X from all nutritional fronts—carbohydrates, fats, protein, and vitamins and minerals—so it works for people with all types of blood-sugar-related conditions, from those who are just a few pounds overweight to those who have full-blown diabetes. We're confident that whatever your age and whatever your state of health, the Anti-X program can turn your health around, too.

Jack Challem, The Nutrition Reporter™
Burton Berkson, M.D., Ph.D.
Melissa Diane Smith, Dipl. Nutr.

ACKNOWLEDGMENTS

As with any book, we have a number of people to thank for their personal and professional contributions to making this project a reality.

We would like to thank Beth Salmon, editor-in-chief of *Let's Live* magazine, who early on saw the potential for a book on Syndrome X and encouraged us to pursue it.

Our appreciation also goes to our agent, Michael Cohn, and to our editor at John Wiley & Sons, Tom Miller, for their commitment to Syndrome X as a book concept. We also thank Shari Dorantes Hatch and Sibylle Kazeroid for their conscientious editing of the manuscript.

We would also like to express our gratitude to Manfred Dunker, Ken Fox, Claus Gehringer, Paul Ross, and Patrick Bridges for their encouragement and their unwavering belief that the message of this book should reach a large audience.

Thanks also to Ken Snyder, Stuart Sandler, Lynn Flance, Holly Sollars, and Don Smith for their support and help with some of the ideas in this book—and a very special thank-you to Helen Smith for her help with recipes and for her careful reading of and comments on the manuscript.

Finally, we would like to acknowledge some of the many people whose original ideas helped shape our thinking on Syndrome X: the late John Yudkin, M.D.; Gerald M. Reaven, M.D.; Robert C. Atkins, M.D.; and Thomas L. Cleave, M.D. We hope this book carries their ideas in expanded form to the general public for a healthier world.

INTRODUCTION

You ARE ABOUT to be engulfed in one of the largest disease epidemics ever to strike North America. It is not a dangerous new flu or some other supergerm. Rather, it is a disorder caused by your body's inability to make the most of the food you eat.

This disorder will age you prematurely, making you feel older than you should. If you have this condition, you will also have a sharply increased risk of practically every age-related disorder, including obesity, hypertension, nervous-system disorders, eye disease, diabetes, cardiovascular disease, cancer, and Alzheimer's disease. In addition to physical symptoms, you may feel exhausted, spacey, depressed, irritable, or angry when you shouldn't be.

Doctors who recognize the underlying cause of this epidemic call it by one of several, often overlapping names: insulin resistance, metabolic syndrome, glucose intolerance, prediabetes, or Syndrome X. In this book, we use the term *Syndrome X*, which includes insulin resistance and one or more related health problems, such as obesity, high cholesterol, high blood pressure, and high triglycerides. Even if you have insulin resistance alone, without the other problems linked to Syndrome X, our cautions and suggestions apply to you. Although few people have recognized the full scope of this disorder, it affects, to one degree or another, the majority of people.

If you are over the age of 35, you may be more familiar with some of the early signs and symptoms than with the names of this condition: feeling sluggish—physically and mentally—after you eat and at many other times, as well; gaining a pound here and a pound there, and having increasing difficulty losing weight; having your blood pressure creep up year after year; and finding that your cholesterol, triglyceride, and blood-sugar levels are doing the same. These are all accepted signs of getting older, but they are all easily reversible.

1

Such symptoms indicate that something is fundamentally wrong with your health, and they have an *additive effect,* meaning that two or three of these symptoms (such as obesity plus high blood pressure) increase your risk of serious disease far more than just one symptom. Look at your own health: Are you a little flabbier than you would like to be, is your blood pressure a little higher than it should be, or is your cholesterol up more than your doctor says it should be? Uncorrected, these symptoms will add up year after year, and their effect will become magnified, undermining your health and all your hopes for a happy and healthy future.

Do you want some *good* news? You have the power within you to turn all of this around. You can reverse these changes and prevent a downward spiral in your life and health. You can spend the rest of your life feeling better, not worse.

We know this is possible because we have seen dramatic improvements in health in ourselves and in other people with Syndrome X who have followed our program. A case in point: A couple of years ago, Jack Challem's fasting glucose was 111 milligrams per deciliter (mg/dl)—high normal and just shy of what doctors would call pre-diabetes. He had also developed a little paunch, another sign of looming health problems. With guidance from physician Burt Berkson, Jack fine-tuned his supplement regimen to include higher doses of the nutrients that help reverse insulin resistance. Following the advice of nutritionist Melissa Diane Smith, he also went on the Anti-X diet plan we describe in this book. In the span of several months, Jack lost 4 inches from his waistline and almost 20 pounds. His fasting glucose dropped 24 points to an ideal 87 mg/dl.

SYNDROME X IN A NUTSHELL

The key underpinning of Syndrome X is *insulin resistance*—a diet-caused hormonal logjam that interferes with your body's ability to efficiently burn the food you eat. Syndrome X occurs when insulin resistance is combined with high levels of blood fats (cholesterol and triglycerides), too much body fat, and high blood pressure. Both insulin resistance and Syndrome X increase your risk of heart disease and diabetes—and many other serious, life-threatening diseases—because they affect, directly or indirectly, virtually every disease process.

Two of the key players in this life-and-death drama affecting you are substances regarded as absolutely essential for health: *glucose* (also known as blood sugar) and the hormone *insulin*. Because of the foods we, as a population, now eat, our bodies' levels of glucose and insulin have gone out of control. Quite simply, we are overdosing on glucose and insulin—and in high doses, both substances accelerate the aging of our bodies and encourage the development of disease.

THE RELATIONSHIP BETWEEN INSULIN RESISTANCE AND SYNDROME X

It is possible to have insulin resistance independently of Syndrome X. However, Syndrome X *always* incudes insulin resistance—that is, elevated insulin production and inefficient glucose metabolism.

Here's why: Excess insulin production promotes increases in blood fats, blood pressure, and obesity. If you have elevated cholesterol or triglycerides, high blood pressure, or abdominal obesity, you almost certainly also suffer from underlying insulin resistance. Therefore, a person with high blood fats, high blood pressure, or obesity almost always has Syndrome X.

Syndrome X is caused primarily by a diet high in refined carbohydrates, which probably include many of your favorite and frequently eaten foods, such as cereals, muffins, breads and rolls, pastas, cookies, doughnuts, and soft drinks. These refined carbohydrates not only raise glucose and insulin to unhealthy levels but also fail to supply the many vitamins, minerals, and vitamin-like nutrients our bodies need to properly utilize these foods.

In other words, nearly all of us have been eating a diet designed for disaster. We have been eating too many bad foods that set the stage for disease and not enough of the good foods that protect us. As a result, our health is being squeezed in the middle.

NUTRITION IS YOUR BEST MEDICINE

One of the problems people face in reversing Syndrome X is perceptual: the long-held belief that food has relatively little to do with the development and progression of disease and the maintenance of health. In contrast, we believe—and are supported with overwhelming scientific evidence—that the quality of our foods has a direct and fundamental bearing on the quality of our health, more so even than the genes we inherit.

In the coming chapters, we explain how the modern diet has set the stage for overdosing on glucose and insulin and for creating

Syndrome X. We describe the baseline diet that people evolved on, how this diet has changed, especially over the past hundred years or so, and how you can easily restore many aspects of traditional diets while still enjoying the food you eat.

We also explain the interplay of diet and physical fitness (through moderate and easily doable activities), and we describe the key supplemental vitamins, minerals, herbs, and vitamin-like nutrients that can be used to jump-start, as well as to fine-tune, your body's defenses against Syndrome X. Chief among these supplements is alpha lipoic acid, a remarkable nutrient that can safely lower glucose and insulin levels. We even give you some very specific guidelines for individualizing the general recommendations of this book, including sample meal plans and nutritional supplement regimens.

The take-home message of this book is relatively simple: You don't have to go through life without a sense of vitality, and you don't have to accept Syndrome X as an inevitable part of an age-related physical decline. We know that you can feel better and reduce your risk of obesity, diabetes, heart disease, cancer, Alzheimer's disease, and other age-related physical and mental disorders. You also won't have to wait years to see the benefits. You will start to see side benefits (instead of side effects) very, very quickly—probably within days of adopting just some of our recommendations.

PART ONE

Syndrome X: The Nutritional Disease

CHAPTER 1

The Food-Health Connection

BY THE TIME Janet Russell of Seattle, Washington, was in her late 30s, her weight had crept up to 245 pounds on her 5′4″ frame, and her blood pressure was a dangerously high 145/95. With her total cholesterol at 240, her "good" cholesterol at a measly 20, and her triglycerides topping out at 250, she was a clear candidate for a heart attack. On top of all this, her fasting glucose (blood-sugar) level was a high 130, so she was also on her way to becoming diabetic.

Laboratory tests, of course, often sound abstract and unreal. After all, you can't *feel* your cholesterol, even if it is high, and most people have trouble relating to diabetes. Janet could feel her deteriorating health on a day-to-day basis, however. Walking up the gentle slope toward her house, she'd get completely winded. It wasn't just the weight she was lugging around; it was the hard work her heart and lungs had to do to move her. By the time she'd get to her doorway, her heart rate would be racing, and her lungs would be huffing and puffing.

The weight would also add drag in other ways. The pounds added pressure to her back, making it ache almost all of the time. As a mother who worked outside the home, Janet went through life in pain and feeling perpetually fatigued. To get the energy she needed at home and at work, she would goose herself with several cups of coffee and four 44-ounce bottles of caffeinated cola on a typical day. The rest of her diet was a mess, too. Almost everything she ate was a variation of pasta.

Janet's doctor certainly recognized that his patient was quickly heading for serious heart disease, diabetes, or both, but he saw her health problems as a disconnected group of symptoms, each to be treated separately. He prescribed a hypertensive drug for blood pressure, a stimulant to help her lose weight, and a "statin" drug to lower cholesterol. Janet never started to feel better, though, and the drugs sometimes created unpleasant side effects that left her feeling even worse. As she turned the corner into her 40s, she saw her father (a diabetic) die, her sister die of a weight-complicated disease, and her brother diagnosed as a diabetic. She figured she would soon be next.

At 47—and still no better in health—Janet happened to read a newspaper article describing a condition her doctor had never mentioned: Syndrome X. When reading the symptoms, she immediately recognized herself, but she was a little unsure of trying the diet "prescription" for this condition that was recommended in the article—a moderately high-protein, low-carbohydrate diet. This was the exact opposite of how she thought she should be eating. However, as Janet contemplated the diet and how she looked and felt, she decided to give the diet a try. Though it was difficult at first to break old habits, Janet slowly but surely phased out the pasta, potatoes, and colas she had become accustomed to consuming.

To her surprise, after just a few days, Janet felt more energetic. After a week, she had lost several pounds without much effort. Pleasantly surprised and encouraged, Janet kept with the diet. She knew she had at last found the answer to her problems.

As Janet's health improved, she began taking vitamin and mineral supplements and began to feel even better. After several months, she felt strong enough to take a beginning aerobics class.

Today, at age 52, Janet enjoys the best health of her life. Her weight is down to 145 pounds—a 100-pound difference that came slowly (a few pounds a month) but with relative ease. Her cholesterol is down to a healthy 176, her triglyceride level has dropped to 73, and her protective (HDL) cholesterol is up to 65. Janet has been off her medications for three years, and her blood pressure is a healthy 120/85. She regularly goes to aerobics classes and now can easily walk up the hill to her house. Janet is healthy, and her cardiovascular and diabetes risk profile is better than the average person's.

Janet didn't just reduce her risk of developing heart disease and diabetes. By effectively dealing with Syndrome X (which we describe in more detail in Chapters 2 and 3), she stemmed a downward spiral in her health. In midlife, Janet is feeling younger, not older. "I feel like a totally new person," she says. "The difference really is like night and day."

THE IMPORTANCE OF DIET

Janet Russell was lucky enough to discover the reason for her health problems—Syndrome X, a set of related health problems, including insulin resistance and one or more other conditions, such as obesity, high blood pressure, high cholesterol, and high triglycerides. Millions of other people, however, still go through life feeling less than their best and, year after year, develop more risk factors for serious diseases. They have no idea that Syndrome X may be the principal cause of their health problems.

What accounts for the emergence of Syndrome X? It is what we now eat. Ironically, it took most of the twentieth century for researchers and physicians to even *start* recognizing that diet is one of the most powerful—and controllable—influences on health and disease. Unbalanced diets are the most common causes of heart disease, cancer, diabetes, and other familiar afflictions. Researchers and physicians are also slowly accepting the fact that Alzheimer's disease, rheumatoid arthritis, mood and behavioral disorders, and countless other health problems are related to the foods we do or do not eat.

To appreciate the importance of diet, you have to recognize that all of the building blocks of your body—the bricks and mortar of your biology, so to speak—come from food. If you eat high-quality foods, you create a strong foundation for health. In contrast, if you fill yourself up on quick and convenient but poor-quality foods, the foundation of your health weakens and you become more vulnerable to disease.

ASSESSING YOUR RISK

Short of undergoing a battery of blood tests, how can you determine whether you may have insulin resistance or Syndrome X? The following two sets of questions, while not entirely scientific, can help you assess your individual risk. In the first quiz, answer all of the questions, then add up the total number of "yes" answers. In the second quiz, check "yes" or "no" to each question, then tally up the points assigned to each "yes" answer. Be honest, so that you can accurately assess your risk.

Diet, Lifestyle, and Risk-Factor Quiz

1. Do you eat sweets—such as candy, cookies, ice cream, pastries, and doughnuts—three or more times a week? ❑ Yes ❑ No

2. Do you eat fat-free foods—such as fat-free muffins, fat-free fruit yogurt, fat-free cookies, or fat-free breakfast bars—more than three times a week? ❑ Yes ❑ No

3. Do you eat potato chips, pretzels, breakfast bars, granola, or ready-to-eat breakfast cereals more than three times a week? ❑ Yes ❑ No

4. Do you eat meals that emphasize pasta, rice, corn, or potatoes more than a couple times a week? ❑ Yes ❑ No

5. Do you eat burgers, hot dogs, fatty luncheon meats (e.g., bologna, ham, salami, pastrami), bacon, sausage, french fries, and fried chicken more than a couple times a week? ❑ Yes ❑ No

6. Do you eat convenience foods (pizza, fast-food-style Mexican food, sandwiches, or snack foods) more than a couple times a week? ❑ Yes ❑ No

7. Do you drink any regular (nondiet) soft drinks? ❑ Yes ❑ No

8. Do you drink more than a small (six-ounce) glass of fruit juice per day? ❑ Yes ❑ No

9. Do you drink more than three beers—or more than a pint of hard liquor—per week? ❑ Yes ❑ No

10. Do you drink more than four glasses of wine per week? ❑ Yes ❑ No

11. Do you avoid regular structured exercise? ❑ Yes ❑ No

12. Are you physically inactive—in other words, do you avoid walking, taking stairs, doing housework, gardening, playing with your children, and so on? ❑ Yes ❑ No

13. Have you had bad eating habits or been a "couch potato" for many years? ❑ Yes ❑ No

14. Do you have a close relative who had or has heart disease, high blood pressure, adult-onset diabetes, or obesity? ❑ Yes ❑ No

If you answered "yes" to more than three questions, you are at risk of developing insulin resistance and Syndrome X—the more "yes" answers, the higher your risk. If you answered "yes" to five or more questions, you need to take immediate action to reduce your risk of developing Syndrome X.

Understanding the questions. Your risk of developing Syndrome X is influenced primarily by what you eat. By consuming many modern foods, as well as having inadequate physical activity, you increase your risk of developing this syndrome. These foods raise the blood levels of both glucose and insulin, setting in motion changes that lead to insulin resistance and Syndrome X.

Symptom Quiz

1. Do you often feel tired, particularly after eating lunch or dinner? ❑ Yes (1 point) ❑ No (0 points)

2. Do you have difficulty concentrating? ❑ Yes (1 point) ❑ No (0 points)

3. Would you characterize your thinking as frequently fuzzy or spacey? ❑ Yes (1 point) ❑ No (0 points)

4. Do you often find yourself irritable or angry? ❑ Yes (1 point) ❑ No (0 points)

5. Do you experience frequent cravings for sugar or other carbohydrates such as pasta, bread, and baked goods? ❑ Yes (2 points) ❑ No (0 points)

6. Do you have a tendency to binge on sweets and other carbohydrates? ❑ Yes (1 point) ❑ No (0 points)

7. Do you feel shaky if you don't eat on time or if you don't snack? ❑ Yes (3 points) ❑ No (0 points)

8. Do you tend to gain weight easily and have difficulty losing it? ❑ Yes (3 points) ❑ No (0 points)

9. Are you overweight, even just 10 pounds over your "ideal" weight? ❑ Yes (3 points) ❑ No (0 points)

10. a. If you're a man, do you have a "pot belly," or a roll, paunch, or "love handles" around your waist? ❑ Yes (5 points) ❑ No (0 points)
    b. If you're a woman, do you carry fat more in the abdominal region or upper body instead of on the hips and thighs? ❑ Yes (5 points) ❑ No (0 points)

11. Do you have high cholesterol levels (above 240 mg/dl), or are you taking medication to control your cholesterol?
❑ Yes (3 points)   ❑ No (0 points)

12. Do you have high triglycerides (above 160 mg/dl)?
❑ Yes (4 points)   ❑ No (0 points)

13. Do you have high blood pressure (consistently above 140/90), or are you taking medication to control your blood pressure?
❑ Yes (5 points)   ❑ No (0 points)

14. Do you feel a need to urinate frequently, or do you often experience unexplained thirst?   ❑ Yes (5 points)   ❑ No (0 points)

15. Have you been diagnosed with either adult-onset diabetes (also known as Type 2 or non-insulin-dependent diabetes) or coronary heart disease?   ❑ Yes (20 points)   ❑ No (0 points)

If your points total between 0 and 3, congratulations—you have minimal risk for insulin resistance and Syndrome X. You're probably doing many things right in your diet and lifestyle, but use this book to learn a little more about how to keep yourself healthy. Also, take this quiz periodically to make sure your risk stays low.

If your points total between 4 and 8, you probably have some degree, or at least the beginning stages, of insulin resistance and possibly Syndrome X. It's important to make the simple diet and lifestyle changes we outline in this book to reverse this trend and reduce your risk of disease.

If your points total between 9 and 19, you probably have insulin resistance and very probably Syndrome X. It's time to take action to nip this process in the bud before your health gets any worse.

If your points total 20 or more, you almost assuredly have Syndrome X. It is imperative that you take strong corrective action with your diet, physical activity level, and the use of supplements. Insulin resistance can be reversed, but you must not wait any longer, or you will continue to see your health deteriorate.

Understanding the questions. Insulin resistance results from the body's inability to deal with large quantities of dietary carbohydrates such as sugars, breads, and pastas. Early signs can include fuzzy thinking and feeling tired after meals. Syndrome X consists of a combination of insulin resistance and one or more of the following problems: upper-body obesity, abnormal blood fats (high cholesterol and high triglycerides), and high blood pressure. Syndrome X greatly increases the risk of heart disease and diabetes, and it also accelerates the aging process.

THE DECLINE OF THE DIET

You may rub your full tummy and believe that you're eating reasonably well, but the odds are, you are not. Most people lack an understanding of how the human diet has changed over the past hundred years or so. During this time, with the merging of traditional agriculture and modern technology, radical changes have occurred in the ways our foods are grown, processed, manufactured, prepared, and consumed. These changes have affected the quality of our food—and our health.

Think about a few of these changes, just for a moment. Do you remember the time before fast-food restaurants, such as McDonald's and Burger King, dotted the landscape—or before microwave ovens made your kitchen the equivalent of a fast-food restaurant? Do you remember when pasta was something eaten only in Italian restaurants—and then only as a special treat?

Do you recall a time before people ate "breakfast bars," a euphemism for sugar-laden breakfast cookies? Do you remember when teenagers drank juice or milk or water instead of cans of cola early in the morning? Can you think back to when you ate home-cooked meals with *fresh* meats and *fresh* vegetables?

It wasn't all that long ago. In the space of little more than a generation, North Americans have adopted major changes in their eating habits. Unfortunately, most of these changes have not been good ones.

Taking a longer view, over the past century, the average person's consumption of refined sugars has increased from several pounds to more than 150 pounds a year. Most of these sugars are added to your food before you buy it. Sugar, in this quantity, wreaks havoc with how your body works and sets the stage for Syndrome X.

Since the mid-1970s, the consumption of refined carbohydrates—pastas, breads, and sweets—has increased by almost 30 percent. This change is partly the result of the popularity of low-fat, high-carbohydrate diets—diets that actually make Syndrome X worse! In addition, dietary fat intake has become totally skewed and abnormal. Indeed, common cooking oils (such as corn and safflower oil) may be the most refined foods people eat, and they often have undesirable druglike effects on health. All of these changes have negative health consequences because our bodies were not designed to handle these highly refined foods.

Unfortunately, when people hear about health problems that involve glucose and insulin, they tend to think only of diabetes, a disease that is out of mind and out of sight for most people. It turns out that nothing could be further from the truth. Excessively high levels of glucose and insulin are common without full-blown diabetes, and they are culprits in a wide variety of health problems. If we want to stay healthy, Syndrome X should *not* be out of sight, out of mind. In the next chapter, we explain what glucose and insulin do and how excessive levels of them damage our health.

CHAPTER 2

Understanding Glucose and Insulin

To BETTER APPRECIATE the problem—Syndrome X—it helps to have an understanding of glucose and insulin and how they interact. *Glucose*, a simple sugar, is also known as blood sugar. It flows through the bloodstream and is the principal fuel of all body cells. Glucose is, in other words, our biological gasoline. *Insulin*, a hormone made by a gland called the pancreas, escorts glucose from the blood into cells, where it is burned for energy.

Levels of glucose and insulin fluctuate a little throughout the day. You can envision glucose and insulin on an axis, much like a playground seesaw. Under ideal circumstances, they move gently and within a limited range, instead of jerking sharply up and down.

GLUCOSE, THE BODY'S FUEL

Your body is composed of about 60 trillion microscopic cells, many of which are highly specialized. Some are heart cells, others are lung cells, and so forth. Although their functions may vary, they all work in similar fundamental ways.

Glucose is burned to power all of these cells. Other biological fuels include glycogen (the form of glucose stored in the liver), amino acids (building blocks of protein), dietary fats, and ketone bodies (made from the breakdown of stored fats).

In terms of sugars, you are probably most familiar with sucrose, or ordinary table sugar, which rapidly breaks down during digestion into equal parts of glucose and fructose. The rapidity of this breakdown is not healthy, as we soon explain.

SOME HELPFUL DEFINITIONS

Glucose. This simple sugar, also known as "blood sugar," fuels each of the 60 trillion cells in your body. Glucose is produced chiefly through the breakdown of carbohydrates (such as sugars) during digestion.

Insulin. This hormone helps shuttle glucose from the blood to the cells. It is also one of the body's most important chemical messengers, telling cells what to do.

Insulin sensitivity (or insulin receptivity). This is the normal and preferable state, in which your body's cells remain sensitive (or receptive), and responsive, to insulin's action.

Hyperinsulinism. This term applies to abnormally elevated levels of insulin in the body. It literally means "high insulin."

Insulin resistance. Abnormally high glucose levels trigger an increase in insulin to remove this sugar from the bloodstream. Often, the body's cells start to ignore high insulin levels and thus become resistant to the hormone's effects. Insulin resistance allows glucose levels to rise and stay high.

Syndrome X. This disorder is characterized by a cluster of associated health problems that together increase the risk of diabetes and coronary heart disease. These problems include having insulin resistance and one or more of the following: glucose intolerance, overweight, abnormal blood fats (e.g., high cholesterol or high triglycerides), and high blood pressure.

Every cell in the body requires a relatively steady supply of glucose to function normally. When glucose levels fall too far or too quickly, cells start to behave like a car sputtering as it runs out of gas. For example, people with severe bouts of low blood sugar (*hypoglycemia*) may become shaky and unsteady. You may sometimes feel a little like this if you do not eat on time.

Humans have complex biological safeguards that protect, at least most of the time, against such dangerous extremes. Hormones are part of the network that signals changes around us and within our bodies. For example, low glucose levels trip a hormonal switch that makes you hungry, prompting you to open the refrigerator door, while the liver temporarily releases glycogen (stored glucose) to boost and normalize glucose levels.

These responses maintain relatively steady glucose levels and keep cells functioning within a normal and optimal range. Normal "fasting" glucose levels—that is, glucose levels when you wake up in the morning—range from 65 to 120 milligrams per deciliter (mg/dl) of blood. The ideal range is 80–100 mg/dl.

After you eat, glucose levels initially rise and then decline slowly. Doctors call this your "postprandial" (postmeal) curve, and the normal peak in this curve is between 65 and 139 mg/dl. Very high fasting and postprandial glucose levels are indicative of diabetes, the condition most often associated with glucose and insulin abnormalities. Moderately high curves may be indicative of prediabetes, or insulin resistance. In contrast, a very modest increase in your postprandial glucose curve indicates very good insulin sensitivity—that is, that your glucose/insulin system is responsive and very well balanced.

INSULIN, THE SUGAR-REGULATING HORMONE

Enter, now, the second player: the hormone insulin, needed for most of the body's cells to properly utilize glucose. Insulin is widely recognized as a "metabolic" or "anabolic" hormone. As a metabolic hormone, it governs a considerable share of *metabolism*—the sum of all the chemical reactions that occur within the body. Seen as an anabolic hormone, insulin plays key roles in the building of new tissue. Insulin's anabolic functions occur chiefly by stimulating cells to take up glucose, which provides the energy to build new tissue. Less well known are insulin's important nonmetabolic hormonal functions (which we describe in the next chapter).

In the 1960s, when researchers learned how to measure insulin levels, they made an amazing discovery. They realized that adult-onset diabetes (also known as Type 2 or non-insulin-dependent diabetes) was more than just a disorder of high glucose levels. It turned out that people with adult-onset diabetes had insulin levels higher than those of nondiabetics. It was a bit of a puzzle, but researchers soon figured out that adult-onset diabetics had become *resistant* to these greater quantities of insulin.

Another hormone that plays a role in glucose management is glucagon, which is also produced by the pancreas. When glucose levels fall, glucagon promotes both the release of glycogen (stored glucose) from the liver and the conversion of protein to glucose.

For all practical purposes, these are stopgap measures because glycogen stores are limited.

By constantly adjusting the secretion of insulin and glucagon—think again of the seesaw—the pancreas and liver work together to maintain relatively steady levels of glucose. These biological methods for controlling glucose developed over millions of years, with mammals—and particularly primates—eating a diverse but relatively simple diet, consisting of protein, carbohydrates, fats, vitamins, and minerals.

All of the carbohydrates eaten were complex in chemical structure and contained within a tough, fibrous matrix, making them only partially digestible—and slowly digested at that. As a result, they prompted a slow, steady increase in glucose and insulin levels—very similar to what happens after a person eats a high-protein, low-carbohydrate meal.

MEASURING GLUCOSE AND INSULIN LEVELS

There are many ways for physicians to assess a person's glucose and insulin levels, as well as insulin resistance. Some of these methods, while very precise, are not very patient friendly. For example, the "euglycemic clamp" technique hooks patients up to intravenous needles. Insulin is infused to a specific level, and this is followed by an infusion of glucose. The physician looks at how much glucose is needed to maintain normal levels.

The more common method involves taking an oral "glucose tolerance test." A patient fasts for some time and then drinks a solution containing 75 grams of glucose. Blood is periodically drawn over a two-hour (or longer) period to determine how high the glucose levels rise and how quickly they fall off.

In a healthy person, glucose levels rise a little, then decrease slowly and sort of plateau out. In a diabetic, glucose levels rise very high and decrease very slowly. Although doctors directly measure changes in glucose, they infer insulin function. A response more typical of a diabetic or prediabetic would be defined as hyperglycemia and would be suggestive of insulin resistance.

A physician might also draw blood to specifically measure insulin levels, though this is not commonly done. For doctors and patients, part of the problem they face with testing is determining what an insurer, such as an HMO (health maintenance organization) will reimburse.

- In general, a normal fasting (morning, before eating or drinking) glucose should be between 65 and 120 mg/dl. An ideal range would be between 80 and 100 mg/dl.
- A normal fasting insulin range is 6–35 micro-international units per milliliter (mcIU/ml).
- A normal two-hour postprandial (postmeal) glucose is generally between 65 and 139 mg/dl.
- A normal two-hour postprandial insulin range is 6–35 mcIU/ml.

INSULIN RESISTANCE: WHEN THINGS GO AWRY

Now consider what happens when you eat highly refined carbohydrates, such as a breakfast bar or doughnut with a cup of sugar-laden coffee, a sandwich on a thick baguette, a bowl of pasta or a couple of slices of pizza, a can of cola, or a convenient microwave dinner.

You overdose on highly refined, rapidly digested carbohydrates and sugars—all of which are quickly converted to glucose. Because large amounts of glucose are toxic to the kidneys and other organs, the pancreas responds by releasing large amounts of insulin to lower the glucose levels. The insulin moves glucose into cells, where it is either burned for energy or stored as fat (triglyceride in adipose cells).

In some people, the pancreas can compensate for a number of years by secreting more and more insulin. These people will appear to be "normoglycemic"—that is, will maintain normal glucose levels and not become overtly diabetic.

In time, though, the body's ability to deal with all this glucose wears out. When people keep consuming large quantities of refined carbohydrates and sugars year after year, skeletal muscle cells (that is, the muscles that wrap around your bones and where most glucose/insulin activity occurs) start to become overwhelmed by all of the insulin, and they start to respond to the insulin much more sluggishly.

Meanwhile, the pancreas keeps receiving signals that glucose levels are high, so it further ratchets up insulin production. The more insulin that's released, the less effective it becomes, and the more resistant to insulin the body's cells become.

Aggravating the situation, insulin also promotes the formation of fat, technically known as *lipogenesis*. In other words, the more insulin a person secretes, the more likely he or she will gain weight!

Without regular physical activity (which burns glucose and lowers insulin levels), insulin keeps increasing the ratio of fat cells to muscle cells. With more fat cells and fewer muscle cells, the body loses still more of its ability to efficiently burn up glucose. Ultimately, both glucose and insulin levels remain elevated—a virtual prescription for Syndrome X, diabetes, and heart disease.

The prevalence of this problem should frighten everyone. According to the recent surveys, 55 percent of all U.S. residents are now overweight—and everyone who is overweight has insulin resistance. In addition, an estimated 25 percent of thin, apparently healthy, nondiabetic U.S. residents also suffer from undiagnosed insulin resistance. In other words, the majority of people—more than 65 percent—suffer from insulin resistance. Similar patterns have occurred as other nations, such as in Europe and Asia, forgo traditional diets in favor of refined foods that boost glucose and insulin levels.

FATS AND CARBOHYDRATES IN THE DIET

Over the years, doctors and public-health officials have tended to focus on health problems resulting from too much dietary fat, not carbohydrates such as sugars. The average person currently eats a diet consisting of about 40 percent fat, and diets high in saturated fat (found in beef) are widely regarded as contributing to coronary heart disease.

High-Fat and Low-Fat Diets

The basic idea behind the "fat is dangerous" idea is that dietary fat deposits on arteries, constricting blood vessels and causing heart disease and heart attacks. As researchers have discovered more about the genesis of heart disease, it has become clear that a blanket "fat is dangerous" view is overly simplistic. Many fats are essential nutrients—without them, we cannot achieve and maintain health. Part of the problem, which we discuss later, relates to a serious imbalance in the types of fats we consume. This is not to say that large quantities of fats are irrelevant. Rather, diets high in the *wrong types* of fat make insulin resistance worse.

Fats are transported through the bloodstream in several principal forms, including cholesterol, triglycerides, phospholipids, and free fatty acids. Free fatty acids are bound to the protein albumin in the bloodstream, and they can be interpreted as a marker of overall fat levels affecting the cardiovascular system.

What makes free fatty acids of particular interest is this: They interfere with the burning of glucose and increase insulin resistance. In a sense, free fatty acids smother the fire that burns glucose. As a consequence, high-fat diets aggravate insulin resistance in healthy subjects, as well as those with obesity or diabetes.

Low Fat Equals High Carbohydrate

So, are low-fat diets an alternative? No.

In recent years, large numbers of people have adopted low-fat diets and regularly eat low-fat or zero-fat foods, in the belief that such diets are healthy and can help them to reduce weight and lower their risk of heart disease. However, low-fat diets are just one more fad in a seemingly endless succession of fad diets.

Low-fat diets typically translate to high-carbohydrate and often high-calorie diets, and their popularity has greatly increased the prevalence of obesity in recent years. In fact, diets high in refined carbohydrates are ideal for promoting insulin resistance and obesity.

In addition, there is compelling evidence showing that people eating low-fat diets have greater feelings of anger, hostility, and depression. These mood changes do not result from psychological feelings relating to dieting. Rather, they appear to be biological consequences of inadequate dietary fat in the central nervous system.

Dietary fat has the attribute of promoting a sense of satiety—leaving a person feeling filled and satisfied from a meal. Without sufficient fat in a meal, most people do not feel satisfied, so they tend to eat more. The "more" in low-fat foods is almost always a larger quantity of refined carbohydrates, which lead to higher glucose and insulin levels and, for many people, an increase in body fat.

Carbohydrate Confusion

Most unrefined, or complex, carbohydrates do not have this excessive glucose- and insulin-stimulating effect. Consumers are not always able to distinguish between refined and unrefined carbohydrates, however, and today they are awash in a sea of highly refined carbohydrates. Contributing to the problem is that the U.S. Department of Agriculture's food pyramid, a key icon of public-health nutrition efforts, fails to distinguish between refined and unrefined carbohydrates. Refined carbohydrates include bakery products, pastas, and sugar-containing foods. Unrefined carbohydrates are found in fruits and vegetables, nuts, and legumes.

Further adding to the problem is the difference in how refined and unrefined carbohydrates are marketed by food companies. Unrefined carbohydrates don't have a lot of marketing pizzazz. The relative lack of marketing and advertising behind them leads to the perception that they may be wholesome, but that they are boring, unappetizing, and unoriginal. Apples and sunflower seeds aren't the object of multimillion-dollar marketing campaigns. The selling of unrefined carbohydrates is usually relegated to low-budget efforts and the "health food" industry, which is an economically small player compared with the giant companies—such as General Foods, Coca-Cola, or Campbell's—that market products high in refined carbohydrates.

In fact, the incentive in business is to design, manufacture (not grow!), and market new food products, and to create new markets for these foods. Sugars and refined grains are extremely pliable, from a manufacturing standpoint, and they lend themselves to what seems a limitless number of new products, including breakfast bars, sugar-drenched cereals, frozen microwavable meals, pizzas, pancakes, soft drinks, confectionaries, and fast-food "value meals" (providing more carbohydrates and sugars for your money!). The bottom line in all this is that *the food industry is geared toward highly processed foods that, by their very nature, promote insulin resistance.*

Add to this dismal dietary picture the fact that insulin resistance tends to increase during normal aging—after all, an older body is by nature less efficient than a younger one. The combination of age and an insulin-resistance-promoting diet exacerbates health problems, such as Syndrome X.

HOPE FOR REVERSING INSULIN RESISTANCE

Can insulin resistance be reversed? Yes—and relatively easily: Insulin resistance results from dietary imbalances, and diet can be easily modified, assuming there is a willingness to avoid some foods and to consume others. Genetics may determine whether you become insulin resistant quickly or slowly, but diet is the principal controllable factor influencing this disorder.

To illustrate the potential for reversing this condition, researchers have found that modest dietary improvements and light exercise led to a 20 percent decrease in insulin resistance in patients. Other studies, which we describe later, demonstrate beyond any doubt that dietary improvements and the selective use of nutritional supplements can greatly improve glucose control, insulin function, and many other aspects of health.

In the next chapter, we explore how insulin resistance forms the cornerstone of Syndrome X, a group of common, associated disorders. We explain how elevated glucose and insulin levels, insulin resistance, and other aspects of Syndrome X accelerate the aging process, and we begin discussing how this process can be halted and reversed.

CHAPTER 3

Syndrome X: Unconnected Symptoms, Connected Causes

SYNDROME X has often been the subject of technical articles in such medical journals as *Hypertension, Diabetes*, and the *American Journal of Epidemiology*. As medical interest in this disorder has grown, information about it has percolated into consumer magazines. Since the late 1990s, such magazines as *Prevention, Let's Live*, and even the conservative *Tufts University Health & Nutrition Letter* have published articles sounding the alarm on this glucose-based disorder.

In this chapter, we explain how insulin resistance forms the core of Syndrome X, which by some estimates affects one in every four adult Americans, as well as adults in other developed nations. We also begin describing how some vitamins and prudent eating play roles in preventing Syndrome X.

THE NATURE OF SYNDROME X

One side effect of specialization is that doctors too often focus only on their area of training and become largely oblivious to what's happening in other medical disciplines. It's the old story of not seeing the forest for the trees. As silly as it sounds, the end result is that doctors often act as though bodies are made of unrelated organs, glands, and limbs. Yet the same blood, carrying the same glucose, hormones, and nutrients, that passes through one organ also flows through every other organ.

24

In theory, specialists (such as cardiologists and endocrinologists) should consult with each other, so they don't lose touch with the bigger picture of a patient's health. Unfortunately, this ideal does not occur as often as we would like. Syndrome X is a case in point. Many doctors treat the individual components of Syndrome X—glucose and insulin disorders, obesity, abnormal blood fats, high blood pressure—but they fail to connect the dots and see the total syndrome.

When the rare scientists or physicians successfully synthesize information from many different disciplines, they tend to stand out for their original and often breathtaking thinking. For instance, after studying insulin resistance for about 20 years at Stanford University, endocrinologist Gerald M. Reaven realized that the disorder sometimes occurred as part of a constellation of related symptoms, which increased the risk of diabetes and coronary heart disease. Instead of seeing a disparate collection of symptoms and risk factors for diabetes and heart disease, he recognized that they were connected.

In 1988, Reaven coined the term "Syndrome X" to define this cluster of symptoms, which includes (1) insulin resistance and glucose intolerance, (2) obesity, (3) blood-fat abnormalities, and (4) hypertension. Reaven continued to research Syndrome X, and his concept of the syndrome has given impetus to additional research by other scientists.

Since that time, the definition of Syndrome X has often become a little more fluid, and many physicians apply it to patients with as few as two of the classic symptoms of the syndrome (e.g., hypertension and obesity). Whatever the technical definition of Syndrome X, the overall pattern remains: Each of the individual components of Syndrome X increases the risk of developing diabetes and heart disease. A combination of two or more of these components of the syndrome has an additive, or cumulative, effect that increases the risk of diabetes and heart disease even more.

The scale of Syndrome X (and its underlying insulin resistance) as a public-health problem sinks in when you consider that glucose intolerance and insulin resistance affect more than half of the population; and that 55 percent of North Americans are overweight, 50 million have elevated cholesterol levels, and 50 million suffer from hypertension. Because of the aggressive marketing and sale of highly processed and refined foods around the world, these conditions are becoming very common in other nations.

Now, let's look at the four principal components of Syndrome X in more detail.

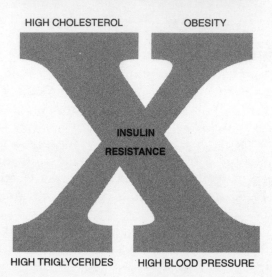

Insulin resistance is the centerpiece of Syndrome X, leading directly or indirectly to the other symptoms associated with Syndrome X. You cannot have Syndrome X without insulin resistance. The original definition of Syndrome X included insulin resistance, obesity, and elevations in cholesterol, triglycerides, and blood pressure. Today, many physicians diagnose Syndrome X when as few as two of the symptoms occur together.

THE SYMPTOMS AND WARNING SIGNS OF SYNDROME X

Syndrome X can be diagnosed when two or more of its related disorders occur simultaneously:

- **INSULIN RESISTANCE AND GLUCOSE INTOLERANCE.** Elevated or erratic levels of glucose, with insulin resistance. Warning sign: fasting glucose above 115 mg/dl.

- **UPPER-BODY OBESITY.** Excess body fat around the stomach or chest. Warning sign: a paunch or "beer belly."

■ **ABNORMAL BLOOD FATS.** Elevated total cholesterol and tri-glycerides and low high-density lipoprotein cholesterol. Warning sign: total cholesterol above 240 mg/dl and triglycerides above 160 mg/dl.

■ **HYPERTENSION.** High blood pressure. Warning sign: consistent blood pressure higher than 140/90.

Insulin Resistance and Glucose Intolerance

Insulin resistance (often along with glucose intolerance and elevated insulin levels) forms the cornerstone of Syndrome X. It is too easy to forget that insulin is one of the body's most powerful *hormones,* a class of chemicals that in very small quantities can produce enormous physical changes. To grasp the power of hormones in general, consider how steroid hormones enhance the muscle mass of body builders, or how estrogen-replacement therapy can change the mental and physical health of women in menopause. Similarly, chronically elevated insulin levels can have a profound effect on health, and we discuss some of its other effects in the next chapter.

Sometimes, instead of frank insulin resistance and chronically elevated insulin levels, people exhibit other forms of glucose intolerance, such as *hypoglycemia* (bouts of low blood sugar). Given the fact that people did not historically eat highly refined carbohydrates, and that the human body is not biologically designed for the glucose "rush" created by such foods, it is not surprising that people easily become intolerant to glucose. It is only normal to be intolerant of something that leads to sickness. The often erratic signs of glucose intolerance indicate that the body simply cannot cope with large loads of refined carbohydrates, and that glucose intolerance is a stepping-stone toward insulin resistance.

The easiest way to diagnose insulin resistance is with a conventional two-hour glucose tolerance test. Typically, a patient drinks a glucose solution, and blood samples (to measure glucose levels) are taken periodically over two hours. Insulin resistance is determined by a glucose curve—that is, a rise and drop in glucose levels—resembling that of a prediabetic (or worse, that of a diabetic). This type of glucose curve rises far above normal and comes down very slowly.

Upper-Body Obesity

Upper-body "apple-type" obesity is a hallmark of Syndrome X. The term is a formal designation for what most people know as a pot belly or a beer belly. Lower-body, pear-shaped obesity (such as fat buttocks) may not be healthy, but it is not generally associated with Syndrome X.

It is important to remember that one of insulin's chief functions is to help the body store fat. In the past, this trait enabled the body to store calories as fat when food was abundant; when food was scarce, the body could draw on these fat reserves. In a society in which food, particularly refined carbohydrates, is plentiful, there is little biological advantage for the body to store fat. Nonetheless, people still carry around fat-storage genes that go into action at a moment's notice. Glucose is stored as fat because it cannot be disposed of any other way (e.g., by burning).

The accumulation of body fat increases the ratio of fat cells to muscle cells. Muscle cells—particularly the skeletal muscle cells in the torso, legs, and arms—are where insulin is most active and where most glucose is burned for energy. People need their muscle cells for all physical movement, such as for walking, jogging, or simply sitting upright and turning the pages of this book. In contrast, fat cells are storage depots that don't burn much of anything.

As the number of fat cells increases, the relative percentage of muscle cells decreases, reducing the number of sites for insulin to function. The situation turns into a vicious cycle, as anyone who has gained weight and tried to lose it knows all too well. As you gain more fat, you have fewer energy-producing muscle cells to devote toward physical activity and the creation of new muscle cells. As time goes on, it becomes more and more difficult to regain the energy, or the psychological motivation, to be more physically active. It's much easier just to be a couch potato. Of course, a lack of physical activity gives insulin all the more opportunity to create still more fat cells.

There is no medical controversy as to whether obesity increases the risk of diabetes and heart disease. Medical experts agree that it does. What's more, the health dangers related to obesity don't stop there. Evidence suggests that obesity also increases the risk of some cancers. For example, obese women are more likely than thin women to develop breast cancer. Similarly, obese people in general have a greater risk of developing cancer of the esophagus. Research may eventually link obesity to many other types of cancer.

A person does not have to be grossly obese to suffer from Syndrome X. As few as 10 pounds of excessive weight can indicate problems, particularly when the extra pounds are also associated with elevated blood fats and high blood pressure. Of course, the more extra weight a person has, the more serious the problem.

Abnormalities in Blood Fats

Cholesterol and triglycerides are the two blood fats most strongly associated with an increased risk of cardiovascular diseases, including heart disease and stroke. However, the cholesterol picture can be extremely complicated and confusing.

Cholesterol is, in fact, an essential substance, and the human body makes most of its own cholesterol in the liver, an organ that functions as our biological chemical-processing factory. All of our steroid hormones, which include testosterone and estrogen, are built around cholesterol. When your skin is exposed to sunlight, your body produces vitamin D from cholesterol. Some researchers believe that increased production of cholesterol and its deposit on the arteries is the body's somewhat misguided attempt at healing injured blood vessels.

In general, physicians view cholesterol as three related entities: total cholesterol, or the sum of all cholesterol in the bloodstream; the "bad" low-density lipoprotein (LDL); and the "good" high-density lipoprotein (HDL). In Syndrome X, a person's total cholesterol level becomes elevated—that is, rises above 240 mg/dl of blood. The bad LDL cholesterol remains within normal levels, but HDL cholesterol, considered the good form of cholesterol, decreases to less than one fourth of the total cholesterol.

At first, all this might sound confusingly contradictory. It turns out that the decrease in HDL cholesterol is significant because it increases the ratio between LDL and HDL, and a high LDL-to-HDL ratio is another risk factor associated with cardiovascular disease. So, a decrease in HDL in Syndrome X is also associated with an undesirable change in the LDL-to-HDL ratio.

BLOOD-FAT PATTERNS IN SYNDROME X

- High total cholesterol levels
- Low HDL cholesterol levels
- High LDL-to-HDL cholesterol ratio
- *Oxidized* LDL cholesterol (damaged by free radicals)
- High triglyceride levels

There's another wrinkle to the cholesterol story. Since the mid-1990s, researchers have noted that "oxidized" LDL cholesterol is more likely to set the stage for heart disease than regular LDL cholesterol. LDL cholesterol is *oxidized*—made rancid, so to speak—by hazardous molecules called *free radicals*. When such damage occurs, white blood cells gobble up the LDL, much as they would do with bacteria. The engorged white blood cells then enter the walls of blood vessels, where they get stuck. As they accumulate, cholesterol deposits develop and narrow the blood vessels, constricting blood flow. One recent study found that oxidized LDL is a characteristic of insulin resistance, which means it is also part of Syndrome X.

Elevated triglyceride levels—above 160 mg/dl—are also associated with Syndrome X and an increased risk of cardiovascular disease. A 1990s study, published in the journal *Circulation*, found that high triglyceride levels were more accurate than elevated LDL cholesterol as a predictor of heart attacks. In fact, people with very high triglyceride levels and very low HDL levels—another pattern characteristic of Syndrome X—are 16 times more likely than normal people to have a heart attack.

To summarize, high total cholesterol, low HDL cholesterol, a high LDL-to-HDL ratio, oxidized LDL, and high triglyceride levels are all part of Syndrome X.

High Blood Pressure

High blood pressure, or *hypertension,* refers to the increased pressure of blood flow within the arteries. It is a serious health problem that, when untreated, can lead to kidney disease, heart disease, and stroke. Hypertension is also associated with memory loss and Alzheimer's disease.

On the surface, increased blood pressure results from one of two causes, or a combination of them: increased pumping force by the heart and a loss of blood-vessel-wall flexibility. Looking deeper, both of these problems can result from many other factors. For example, a heart has to pump harder than normal to push blood through an obese body, and that effort increases blood pressure.

In addition, age-related hardening of the arteries reduces the flexibility of blood vessels. Healthy, young blood vessels can *dilate,* or expand in diameter, as they adapt to different physiological situations and temporary increases in blood pressure, such as during physical exertion or periods of psychological stress. With age, however, blood vessels tend to harden and their openings become narrower, further restricting blood flow and increasing blood pressure.

Diets high in saturated fat and refined carbohydrates also reduce the ability of blood vessels to dilate flexibly, and this effect
can occur within minutes of eating a high-fat meal. One recent
study demonstrated this effect after subjects ate a high-fat, high-
carbohydrate McDonald's breakfast.

The difference between normal and abnormal blood-vessel flexibility is comparable to the difference in the water flow in a three-
quarter-inch garden hose versus a half-inch hose. Given equal water
pressure at the source, water moves through the narrower garden
hose much faster and with much greater pressure than it does
through the wider hose. In other words, large, flexible blood vessels are better for maintaining normal blood pressure.

There is considerable scientific research showing that elevated
glucose and insulin levels, as well as insulin resistance, are common causes of hypertension. Insulin can increase blood pressure in
numerous ways. For example, the hormone can increase the retention of sodium, which raises blood pressure in many people.

Insulin also turns on the body's sympathetic nervous system,
the part of the body's nervous system that speeds up the heart rate
and raises blood pressure. In addition, the hormone increases
secretion of *cortisol*, a stress hormone that constricts blood vessels
and is strongly associated with heart disease and other degenerative diseases. Not surprisingly, a combination of stress and a diet
high in refined carbohydrates can boost blood pressure.

Incidentally, high levels of cortisol are also associated with low
levels of dehydroepiandrosterone (DHEA), a hormone that is commonly depressed in insulin resistance. DHEA is the hormone necessary for production of testosterone, estrogen, and other steroid
hormones and has been reported to have an antiaging effect on
elderly men. It also increases muscle mass, which would improve
the burning of glucose and reduce insulin resistance.

People with hypertension also tend to have faster resting heart
rates. This is another example of how hearts tend to work harder
in people with hypertension. One recent study of 45 healthy
subjects found that high insulin levels and insulin resistance
increased nighttime heart rates. In this study, the researchers used
an oral glucose tolerance test to raise insulin levels and to temporarily induce insulin resistance. Many people unwittingly con-
duct similar experiments at home and at work, because a can of
cola and a fudge brownie are roughly equivalent to a glucose tolerance test.

SYNDROME X RESEARCH

From a scientific standpoint, it can be difficult to demonstrate that a cluster of several conditions are related and, as a group, also sharply increase the risk of diabetes and coronary heart disease. The reason for this difficulty relates to the large number of variables a researcher must track and correlate. For example, it's relatively easy to build a case arguing that obesity increases the risk of diabetes and heart disease. It's much more difficult to argue that cholesterol, triglyceride, obesity, insulin resistance, and hypertension together are commonly associated and increase the risk of diabetes and coronary heart disease.

Some people might criticize Syndrome X as being little more than a group of associated symptoms, without any direct proof that they form a true syndrome that increases the risk of disease. However, savvy health professionals recognize that the clusters of symptoms indicative of Syndrome X are very common. For example, people who are obese are always insulin resistant. Obese people are also more likely than thin, non-insulin-resistant people to develop diabetes or heart disease. Likewise, people with high blood pressure are frequently insulin resistant and often obese. In addition, hypertensive individuals are more likely than nonhypertensive individuals to develop heart disease.

In an illustrative study, researchers at Stanford University investigated the additive effects of high blood pressure, obesity, and adult-onset diabetes (indicative of severe glucose intolerance and insulin resistance) in both thin and obese men and women. The thin subjects with normal blood pressure had the lowest glucose and insulin levels, indicative of normal glucose tolerance and insulin function. In contrast, both thin and obese subjects with high blood pressure had abnormally elevated glucose levels. The worst glucose intolerance and insulin resistance occurred in people who were obese and who also had high blood pressure and diabetes.

DIABETES: THE WORST FORM
OF INSULIN RESISTANCE

Why, you might be wondering, do we keep returning to diabetes as a principal consequence of insulin resistance and Syndrome X? After all, insulin resistance does not always lead to diabetes, and you probably have not been diagnosed as a diabetic. In fact, the whole thought of diabetes may be the furthest thing from your mind.

THE DIABETES CONTINUUM

Glucose Intolerance → Insulin Resistance → Syndrome X → Diabetes

Diabetes is part of a continuum of diseases caused by the excess consumption of refined carbohydrates. Because most people nowadays consume diets filled with highly refined foods, most people are prediabetic to some degree. The early signs of diabetes are glucose intolerance, insulin resistance, and Syndrome X.

Even if you are not diabetic, there are several reasons why you should be concerned about diabetes or, at the very least, about prediabetic symptoms. The first is that diabetes and all other degenerative diseases develop slowly, over years, meaning that various degrees of prediabetes may exist for years. In other words, diabetes is not an all-or-nothing disease, and insulin resistance and Syndrome X are common forms of prediabetes.

The early signs of diabetes are easy to overlook because the symptoms are often vague, and ambiguous symptoms can indicate almost any disorder. Most doctors are taught that diseases have well-defined causes that respond to well-defined treatments. While this idea seems straightforward enough, it has a built-in defect. Diseases are most easily diagnosed in their later stages, not in their earlier stages. Unfortunately, treating diseases in their later stages is often a difficult, uphill battle. It is much easier to prevent disease or to change the course of the illness before the damage becomes entrenched and irreversible. If you know that glucose intolerance and insulin resistance are potentially early signs of diabetes or heart disease, you can correct them before you become diabetic or have a heart attack.

EARLY SIGNS OF ADULT-ONSET DIABETES

- Frequent urination
- Frequent thirst
- Excessive hunger
- Unexplained weight gain
- Inability to concentrate
- Unexplained drowsiness
- Feeling tired most of the time, particularly after lunch or dinner
- Decreased endurance during physical exertion and exercise
- Fasting (morning) glucose levels above 130 mg/dl

Earlier Diagnoses of Diabetes

Another reason for being concerned about diabetes relates to a rapid and frightening increase in its prevalence. Diabetes is more common than you might think. More than 15 million North Americans have diabetes, many without knowing it. Furthermore, more diagnoses of diabetes are being made in people who are younger and younger.

In fact, the situation is rapidly deteriorating. Years ago, the only form of diabetes that children had to fear was juvenile-onset diabetes, in which the pancreas stopped making insulin. Recent newspaper articles have noted the alarming emergence of adult-onset diabetes—the insulin-resistant form of the disease—in obese children. This trend is a sign that the modern diet is rapidly getting worse, and that the health of children is being derailed because they begin eating a diabetes-inducing diet as infants and toddlers—earlier than has any other generation.

The disease-promoting effect of contemporary, highly refined foods is having a clear effect on the "baby boomer" generation, as well. In June 1997, the federal government recommended that all adults be tested for diabetes by the time they reach age 45, before diabetic complications (e.g., heart, kidney, eye, and nerve disease) progress and become difficult to treat. That same month, the American Diabetes Association lowered the bar for diagnosing diabetes. The old standard was a fasting blood sugar of 140 mg/dl or higher; the new standard is 126 mg/dl.

As it turns out, testing people at age 45 may be too late. A survey by Roper Starch Worldwide, released in January 1998, found that baby boomers are being diagnosed with diabetes at the average age of 37, compared with older adults, who were on average 54 years old when they were diagnosed with the disease. In November 1998, researchers from the federal Centers for Disease Control (CDC), in Atlanta, recommended that people should be tested for adult-onset diabetes at age 25!

Diabetes as a Model of Accelerated Aging

Yet another reason to be concerned about diabetic and prediabetic symptoms may be the most significant in terms of maintaining excellent health through midlife and as you enter old age: Many researchers see diabetes as a model of accelerated aging. Diabetics have for years been known to develop various risk factors, symptoms, and diseases earlier than do nondiabetics. For example, diabetics generally develop higher cholesterol levels years before nondiabetics do, and they generally die of heart disease at younger ages, compared with nondiabetics.

Basically, diabetics get old faster than nondiabetics, and it is reasonable to assume that people with elevated (but prediabetic) glucose, insulin resistance, and Syndrome X also age much faster than people without these conditions. From a scientific standpoint, diabetes gives researchers an opportunity to study the aging process in a shorter period of time. From the standpoint of public health, diabetes and Syndrome X are aging the population at a faster pace and making them susceptible to age-related diseases earlier in life.

Why Diabetics Age Faster Than Other People

Why do diabetics age faster than other people? There are a number of reasons, which we briefly describe here and explore in more detail in the next chapter. Elevated glucose generates large numbers of destructive *free radicals,* molecules that damage cells and age them, setting the stage for virtually every degenerative disease.

In addition, glucose generates "advanced glycation end-products," abbreviated as AGEs. AGEs are created by free radicals and damage the protein in cells, preventing them from functioning normally. For example, both free radicals and AGEs damage the eye lenses and cause cataracts, which diabetics have an above-average risk of developing. The same process occurs in the body's other cells.

The point to remember is that aging is the accumulation of damaged cells. When aged cells outnumber younger cells, serious disability or death results. High glucose (and insulin) levels speed up the damage. It's much better to maintain normal glucose levels.

ONE TYPE OF INSULIN-SENSITIVE DIET

In contrast to the age-accelerating effects of excessive carbohydrate consumption and diabetes, caloric restriction has the opposite effect: It leads to greater insulin sensitivity (that is, better insulin function), which is desirable, and extends life span. Research going back more than 60 years clearly demonstrates that eating fewer calories improves health and lengthens life span. Don't worry, though—we are not going to ask you to starve yourself in the name of health. Extreme caloric restriction is not practical for most people, and many of the same health benefits can be achieved through more moderate dietary changes and supplements (which we describe later in this book).

Laboratory studies have consistently found that rodents live about one third longer when their caloric intake is restricted by about 30 percent from birth. Furthermore, experiments have demonstrated that calorie-restricted rodents stay younger physiologically; remain more energetic, mentally sharp, and adaptable; and retain better-looking coats. Translated into human terms, a 50-year-old person who ate a calorie-restricted diet from birth would look and act as youthful as a 33-year-old.

Of course, rats and mice that live for three to four years are very different from people who routinely live into their 70s. A closer relative to humans is the rhesus monkey. Two ongoing studies of caloric restriction in rhesus monkeys, one at the National Institute of Aging and the other at the University of Wisconsin, are already finding that calorie-restricted diets are helping the animals maintain more youthful bodies and minds, compared with monkeys allowed to eat as much as they want.

The monkeys, which are currently entering midlife, are the equivalent of baby boomers. Those eating calorie-restricted diets (with normal levels of vitamins and minerals) have substantially lower blood levels of glucose and insulin, lower levels of total cholesterol and triglycerides, higher levels of the protective HDL form of cholesterol, and substantially lower blood pressures.

In addition, the calorie-restricted monkeys show no signs of diabetes, heart disease, or other age-related diseases, whereas the animals eating regular diets have age-related diseases comparable to middle-aged people. The calorie-restricted monkeys have no insulin resistance or Syndrome X, and they are as healthy as young monkeys.

Again, many of the health benefits of calorie restriction can be achieved through dietary modifications that involve eating more nutrient-dense foods, fewer refined carbohydrates, and a better balance of fats. In addition, supplements, such as alpha lipoic acid (which we discuss later in the book), can safely lower glucose and insulin levels and retard age-related, glucose-dependent damage to the body.

THE SECRET OF LIVING TO AGE 100

The discussion of diabetes and calorie restriction brings us to a 1990s study on *centenarians*—people who live past 100 and, particularly, remain healthy and active. The study revealed some of the physical and dietary traits of people who live past 100 in good health, with lessons relevant to preventing Syndrome X.

Physician Giuseppe Paolisso and his colleagues at the University of Naples, Italy, compared the clinical characteristics—blood chemistries, lifestyle habits, and diets—of three groups of people: healthy adult men and women averaging 40 years old, randomly selected elderly subjects between 70 and 99 years old, and centenarians. Overall, the centenarians were in better health than folks in the 70–99 age group, despite more than a 30-year difference in age among some of the participants.

The centenarians were trimmer, had less body fat, and were less likely to have pot bellies than either the 40-year-olds or the 70- to 99-year-olds. They had lower fasting glucose levels and lower free-fatty-acid levels than either of the other two groups. Their insulin function—based on their ability to remove glucose from the blood—was far superior to that of the 70- to 99-year-olds and virtually the same as that of the 40-year-olds. In other words, the centenarians had few signs of insulin resistance.

What was the secret of their longevity and remarkable health? Paolisso noted that the centenarians suffered less "oxidative stress"—that is, their bodies had fewer dangerous free radicals. They also had higher blood levels of vitamins E and C and glutathione, all antioxidant nutrients that protect against free radicals. These antioxidants limit the production of free radicals and AGEs, including those generated by glucose. The centenarians' diets seemed to make all the difference. They ate about two and one-half times more vegetables—which are foods that are low in carbohydrates and richest in antioxidants—than did the 70- to 99-year-olds and five times the vegetables of the 40-year-olds.

Perceptive as it is, the limitation of Reaven's Syndrome X concept, and even that of insulin resistance per se, is the contention that these diseases essentially relate to one dietary change—namely, the increased consumption of refined carbohydrates. In the next chapter, we go beyond Syndrome X to describe other ways that high levels of glucose and insulin derail health. We also tell you more about how glucose ratchets up the production of dangerous free radicals and AGEs, affecting your ability to resist heart disease, cancer, infections, and many other diseases.

We start to explain how the same diet that induces Syndrome X is also virtually devoid of many vitamins, minerals, and other micronutrients crucial for health. As you read on, you'll discover that the nutritional deficiencies resulting from modern eating habits seriously compromise our ability to cope with refined carbohydates and further exacerbate our health problems.

CHAPTER 4

Beyond Syndrome X: Sugar and Insulin Overload

ALTHOUGH GLUCOSE and insulin form the underpinnings of Syndrome X—and associated diseases—these two substances have far more widespread and hazardous effects on your health than just their role in this disease. High levels of both glucose and insulin, separately and in combination, accelerate the speed at which your body ages and make you susceptible to age-related degenerative diseases earlier in life.

In a nutshell, the choice you face in eating is this: A diet high in sugars and other refined carbohydrates, which boosts glucose and insulin levels, can make you feel older when you're still relatively young; in contrast, a diet low in these foods can help preserve and restore many aspects of youthfulness—and help you resist disease.

In this chapter, we explain the far-reaching and hazardous effects that dietary sugars and overproduction of insulin have on your health. We also start to explain how the modern diet poses a double-whammy to your health, in that it contains excessive amounts of refined carbohydrates *and* inadequate amounts of vitamins, minerals, and other micronutrients needed to properly manage those carbohydrates.

THE SUGAR SYNDROME

Quite simply, sugar and related caloric sweeteners (e.g., high-fructose corn syrup) are some of the most dangerous substances you can put into your mouth.

At first, this idea may seem incomprehensible. Sugar tastes *so* good and leaves you feeling *so* good. Also, in one form or another, it is added to virtually every prepared food. If you read the ingredients list on packaged foods, you will discover how omnipresent sugar is. It is even added to salt!

In general, sugar is defined as *sucrose*, the white crystalline stuff you add to your coffee and use when baking cookies. During digestion, sucrose breaks down into equal parts of glucose and fructose. The glucose half becomes blood sugar; the fructose half causes its own mischief, which we describe shortly.

Since the mid-1980s, high-fructose corn syrup has replaced about half of the sugar added to commercial food products, such as soft drinks, packaged foods, and many baked goods. Although the fructose in the name hints at a natural product—after all, fructose is widely considered "fruit sugar"—it does not come from fruit. It is nothing less than a highly refined and manufactured food product.

High-fructose corn syrup is actually a blend of 55 percent fructose and 45 percent glucose—almost the same ratio as what sucrose yields during digestion. From a food-manufacturing standpoint, high-fructose corn syrup appeals to companies because it is easier to use, less expensive, and has a longer shelf life than conventional sugar. It also tastes much sweeter than sucrose.

Historically, people rarely consumed any kind of refined sugars, other than occasionally eating a bit of honey, which is so sweet that it is difficult to consume much of it. Traditionally, most sweet-tasting foods were consumed in the form of fruits, the sugars of which are part of a matrix that greatly slows their digestion. Later, small quantities of sugar became popular among royalty and monied families—it was just too expensive for the average person.

Over the past couple hundred years, with changes in food processing, sugar consumption began to increase. The estimated per-capita consumption by U.S. residents in the early 1800s was 12 pounds per year. Today, it is more than 150 pounds per year. Similar trends in sugar consumption have occurred in other nations when people have shifted from traditional diets to modern refined ones. Bear in mind, as well, that these numbers are averages, and some people consume less and others more. Statistically speaking, for every person who consumes only 5 pounds of sugar a year, there's another who eats 295 pounds a year.

The consumption of such huge quantities of sugar would be serious if for no other reason than because this food product provides only empty calories and displaces more nutrient-dense foods, such as protein and complex carbohydrates. Soft drinks are a case in point. When your body is thirsty, it needs water, not sugar. What it gets, though, is sugar water. The Center for Science in the Public Interest, based in Washington, D.C., has described soft drinks as "liquid candy." A typical can of soft drink contains about 10 teaspoons of sugar or high-fructose corn syrup, and the average person today consumes 53 gallons of soft drinks a year—double what she or he did in the mid-1970s.

As it is in soft drinks, most sugar or high-fructose corn syrup is added to foods before you even sit down to eat. A 2.1-ounce Three Musketeers bar contains 40 grams of sugars; three quarters of a cup of Kellogg's Frosted Flakes contains 13 grams; a cup of Snapple lemonade contains 27 grams; and a large McDonald's vanilla shake contains 71 grams of sugars. It may sound strange, but sugarholics essentially go through life having the equivalent of several glucose tolerance tests every day!

In the pages that follow, we describe some of the many ways that glucose and insulin age you and make you feel and look worse than you should.

Glucose, Free Radicals, and Aging

After sugars and other refined carbohydrates are broken down in the digestive tract, the glucose portion enters cells, where it is burned for energy. The specific burning process occurs in what scientists call the Krebs cycle. Through numerous steps, glucose is converted into other energy-containing compounds, such as adenosine triphosphate (ATP).

The process is a little like a snowball getting larger and larger as it rolls downhill. The energy from glucose and its derivative compounds is carried by subatomic particles called electrons. As these electrons are passed along a chain of chemical compounds, free radicals and antioxidants are formed. Momentum increases in the form of chemical energy up to the creation of ATP. It is the release of ATP, the end-product of glucose metabolism, that creates energy, which is used to power the cells of your heart, brain, muscles, and other organs.

Free radicals, however, can be highly unstable and destructive. The process of burning, or oxidizing, glucose has a built-in containment that limits the leakage of free radicals outside of the energy-producing chemical reactions. The containment is so efficient that more than 99.99 percent of electrons are confined within these chemical reactions. Nonetheless, the small number of free radicals that do leak out cause cumulative damage to cells and tissues. Over many years, the damage from these free radicals ages our bodies and makes us more susceptible to age-related diseases.

Free radicals cause damage because they are lopsided molecules that lurch around clumsily. Normal molecules contain pairs of electrons. A free radical is missing one electron from that pair. As a consequence, the free radical tries to find a replacement electron as quickly as possible, and it does this by stealing an electron from another molecule. Free radicals are completely indiscriminate, and any molecule will suffice. A free radical that robs an electron from a molecule of deoxyribonucleic acid (DNA, the material that makes up your genes) can mutate, or damage, that DNA. Free-radical damage to DNA is a major cause of aging and cancer.

A SIMPLIFIED LOOK AT GLUCOSE, FREE RADICALS, AND AGING

- When glucose is burned, a lot of energy (ATP) and a small number of free radicals are produced.
- High-carbohydrate diets generate large numbers of free radicals, which deplete the body's antioxidant reserves.
- Excess free radicals damage DNA, and low levels of antioxidants derail the body's natural protective mechanisms.

Two 1990s studies illustrate how glucose increases free radicals in the body. In one, researchers noted that after diabetics ate a meal, the diabetics' levels of free radicals increased, and their levels of some antioxidant vitamins (which neutralize free radicals) decreased. Because of the timing of these changes, the researchers were able to conclude that the high postmeal glucose levels caused the increase in free radicals.

This increase in free radicals, by the way, is often referred to as "oxidative stress," because oxygen molecules are often involved in the creation of free radicals. (Just as your car needs oxygen to burn gasoline, your body needs oxygen to burn glucose.) However, glucose is quite capable of auto-oxidizing—in effect, igniting itself and generating lots of dangerous free radicals.

In the second study, levels of antioxidant vitamins in healthy and diabetic patients dropped significantly after they were given a standard glucose tolerance test. The sudden decrease in antioxidants, including vitamins E and C, was the result of glucose-generated

free radicals suddenly overwhelming the patients' antioxidant reserves. The implications of this study are profound. First, foods
containing a lot of sugar generate huge numbers of free radicals, a
situation that is biologically similar to being exposed to radiation,
cigarette smoke, or air pollution (which also generate large numbers of free radicals). Second, such diets greatly increase the need
for antioxidant vitamins to compensate, at least partly, for all of the
free radicals and to reduce the oxidative stress.

Glucose, AGEs, and Aging

As we mentioned earlier, glucose can also react with and damage
the body's proteins, which form organs and all other tissues. The
by-products of these reactions include AGEs. Basically, glucose
fuses with protein, damaging your body much the way that over-
cooking toughens a steak. Wrinkled skin is one example of the age-
accelerating effect of AGEs.

A SIMPLIFIED LOOK
AT GLUCOSE AND AGEs

High Glucose Reacts with Proteins in Cells

Advanced Glycation End-products (AGEs) Form

AGEs Age Cells

Aged Cells Are More Prone to Disease

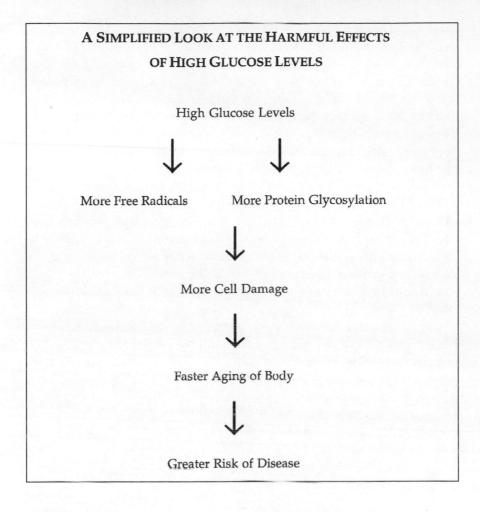

A SIMPLIFIED LOOK AT THE HARMFUL EFFECTS OF HIGH GLUCOSE LEVELS

High Glucose Levels

More Free Radicals   More Protein Glycosylation

More Cell Damage

Faster Aging of Body

Greater Risk of Disease

AGEs contribute to heart disease in a couple of ways. They increase the oxidation of LDL cholesterol, which is one of the earliest steps in the development of heart disease. They also create cross-links in the proteins forming blood-vessel walls, which age those walls and make them less flexible. Free radicals increase the production of AGEs, and some research indicates that free radicals and AGEs kill brain cells.

Although high levels of glucose accelerate the formation of both free radicals and AGEs, high levels of fructose (the other half of common dietary sugars) appear to exaggerate the effect. In an animal study reported in the *Journal of Nutrition,* high-fructose diets raised cholesterol and AGE levels much more than did glucose. We explain more about fructose shortly.

Sugar, Glucose, and Heart Disease

In the 1960s, the late physician and researcher John Yudkin began noticing a relationship between the intake of common dietary sugar (sucrose) and the risk of heart disease. Research since then has confirmed that sugar is *atherogenic*—that is, it causes heart disease. In addition to increasing levels of blood fats, such as blood triglycerides and the LDL-to-HDL ratio, sugar actually makes *blood-platelet cells*—the specific type of cells that form blood clots—stickier and more likely to clump together. Sticky platelets are more likely to clot abnormally in blood vessels, and by doing so, they increase the risk of heart disease and stroke.

The evidence of sugar's effect on platelet stickiness, known as *platelet aggregation,* comes from several lines of observation and research. For one, diabetics are more prone than nondiabetics to having blood clots, particularly the "microvascular" clots that contribute to eye disease and also underlie all cardiovascular disease. Elevated glucose levels, and possibly elevated insulin, as well, increase the production of *thromboxane,* one of the body's blood-clot-triggering compounds. It is also possible that glucose-generated free radicals simply overwhelm the body's antioxidant reserves. For example, diabetic patients with low vitamin E levels are more likely to have very sticky platelets than other diabetics.

HOW HIGH GLUCOSE INCREASES THE RISK OF HEART DISEASE

- It increases triglyceride and the LDL-to-HDL cholesterol levels.
- It makes blood platelet cells stickier, increasing the likelihood of blood clots.
- It generates free radicals that stimulate the overgrowth of smooth-muscle cells, which narrow blood vessels and make clots more likely.

Glucose increases the risk of heart disease in yet another way. The proliferation of "smooth-muscle cells" in blood vessels (not just the building up of cholesterol) contributes to the vessels' narrowing, thereby constricting blood flow. It turns out that glucose-generated free radicals stimulate the growth of smooth-muscle cells in blood vessels.

In addition, a study conducted at the Harvard University School of Public Health found that, among women ages 38–63, consumption of higher quantities of refined carbohydrates increased the risk of heart attacks by 40 percent, compared with women eating smaller amounts of refined carbohydrates. The researchers measured carbohydrate intake using the "glycemic index," which we describe in more detail in Chapter 7.

Glucose and Immunity

Eating sugar also reduces the body's ability to fight infections. In 1908, researchers noted that diabetics were more susceptible than nondiabetics to infection. It took researchers until 1942 to discover that the bacteria-engulfing white blood cells of diabetics were essentially sleeping on the job.

Subsequent studies confirmed that high concentrations of glucose reduce the ability of white blood cells to capture bacteria. For example, researchers at Loma Linda University, California, found that white blood cells from people who ate the equivalent of a candy bar and a soft drink could capture only one tenth of the bacteria, compared with people who ate only half of a candy bar. The reduced immune responsiveness occurred within only 45 minutes, meaning that sugar greatly reduces a person's ability to fight infections. Other research has found that dietary sugars reduce white-blood-cell activity by 50 percent, with the effect lasting for five hours—more than enough time for the average person to have another hit of immune-depressing sugar.

In similar experiments, researchers at Utah State University, Logan, tested the effect of different diets on antibody production in laboratory rats. *Antibodies* are very complex immune compounds designed to combat specific bacteria and viruses. The researchers found that as little as a 10 percent decrease in the nutritional quality of the diet (e.g., 10 percent more sugar and 10 percent less protein, vitamins, and minerals) decreased antibody production by 50 percent. When the amount of sugar in the diet was increased to 75 percent and other nutrients decreased to 25 percent, antibody production dropped by 90 percent. Such changes, in people, would greatly increase susceptibility to infection—and chronic infection increases the risk of heart attack and cancer.

Glucose and Cancer

Although the exact relationship between glucose (and other sugars) and cancer is equivocal, some suggestive evidence does link the two. Cells can grow in two ways: one in sheer size, and the other in number. Whenever cell numbers increase, other than during normal growth or healing processes, the specter of cancer emerges. A couple of studies have found that the risk of biliary cancer (i.e., cancer of the gallbladder's bile ducts) increases with consumption of glucose and sucrose. Also, some researchers have found that a high-sugar diet increases the risk of lung cancer by 55 percent.

The Health Hazards of Fructose

Many people believe that fructose is a healthy alternative to common table sugar, but there are plenty of reasons to avoid fructose, as well. To begin with, the fructose found in food products today doesn't come from fruit; it's a highly refined product from corn, and there are a number of deleterious health effects attributed to its use.

When Yudkin was researching the health effects of sugar (sucrose), he noticed that fructose alone magnified nearly all of the effects found with sucrose. The irony in this is that fructose is considered a safe sugar for diabetics because it does not trigger a rapid rise in blood sugar.

Fructose does, however, do a lot of other things, such as increase free-radical production, boost blood levels of cholesterol and triglycerides, and stimulate the production of insulin and cortisol. Also, despite the fact that fructose does not produce a significant increase in glucose levels, it does promote insulin resistance. One 1990s study found that the addition of fructose to a fat-containing meal—think of a fructose-sweetened cola washing down a cheeseburger—substantially raised postmeal levels of triglycerides.

Fructose can even increase the likelihood of developing osteoporosis. Forrest H. Nielsen and David B. Milne of the USDA's Agricultural Research Service in Grand Forks, North Dakota, placed a group of men on a diet that included five cans of decaffeinated soda (to eliminate any caffeine-related effects) sweetened with high-fructose corn syrup each day. The high-fructose soft drinks reduced the men's levels of calcium and phosphorus, which are needed for healthy bones. The effects of fructose were amplified when the men were also placed on a magnesium-deficient diet. Magnesium intake among people consuming refined diets is marginal because most people do not eat many magnesium-rich foods, such as leafy greens, nuts, and whole grains.

Bizarre as it may sound, a new line of beverages and bars for diabetics is marketed as "healthy snacks that help improve glucose control." Their labels promise to provide balanced and complete nutrition—yet the first ingredient is high-fructose corn syrup!

INSULIN OVERLOAD

Hazardous as sugar is, elevated levels of insulin are an equal partner in metabolic crime. Insulin, of course, is a hormone, a member of a group of chemicals that, in infinitesimally small amounts, exert powerful effects on our bodies. Hormones make some people masculine and others feminine, some people strong and muscular and others weak, some people tall and others short. They also signal changing conditions in the environment surrounding us, as well as within our body, prompting quick adaptive responses. For example, adrenaline can give us the strength to face danger or to run swiftly from it.

Insulin resistance and Syndrome X—and the consequential cascade of disorders—are the result, in large part, of excessive insulin production. What distinguishes insulin from other hormones is that *you don't have to take pills to create abnormally high levels of it.* All you have to do is *eat the typical modern diet,* containing large amounts of sugar and other refined carbohydrates that promote insulin production.

A number of studies have found that elevated insulin levels typically precede, by years, the elevated glucose levels characteristic of diabetes. In addition, glucose intolerance and insulin resistance precede overt heart disease by 8–20 years. The reason may be that because of the way people eat, the pancreas is primed to overreact to refined carbohydrates. In fact, a study at the University of Toronto found that insulin levels increased more sharply than glucose levels after healthy, thin subjects were given carbohydrates.

High levels of glucose undoubtedly trigger an abnormal elevation of insulin, but as long as the pancreas can successfully secrete insulin to compensate for large amounts of glucose, glucose levels will remain within a normal range. The early elevation of insulin, while normal glucose levels are maintained, suggests that many of the health problems stemming from insulin resistance are specifically the result of insulin, not glucose.

Insulin and the Heart

Your skeletal muscle cells are the principal site where insulin and
glucose interact. As the term suggests, these muscle cells surround
your skeleton—your arms, legs, and torso. As glucose is burned,
your muscle cells gain the energy to move, much the way your car
uses gasoline as its source of energy.

Over the years, however, doctors have generally overlooked the
most important muscle in your body: your heart. It has only been
recently that researchers have considered how insulin affects glucose uptake by the heart and how insulin per se influences heart
function.

Just as skeletal muscle cells become insulin resistant, it is conceivable that the heart muscle (also known as the *myocardium*) can
also become insulin resistant, reducing the heart's ability to burn
glucose for energy. Whatever the mechanism, insulin is hazardous
to the heart. Patients receiving insulin therapy have an increased
risk of coronary heart disease, and the amount of insulin injected
on a daily basis is a strong indicator of the degree of risk. Furthermore, ischemic heart disease (a common form of heart disease) is
strongly associated with high levels of insulin in the blood.

Whether or not insulin leads to insulin resistance in heart cells,
the hormone does affect the heart in many other ways. Insulin
alters the behavior of *endothelial cells*, which line artery walls and affect the behavior of blood vessels. Oxidized (free-radical-damaged)
LDL cholesterol—which is associated with insulin resistance—in-
jures endothelial cells, either by damaging them directly or by overwhelming them with free radicals.

Insulin and Stress

Other hormones may also influence insulin levels and insulin resistance. For example, glucocorticoid hormones, made by your
adrenal glands, reduce the ability of insulin to carry glucose into
cells. The principal glucocorticoid hormone is cortisol, which
boosts glucose levels. Cortisol is also considered the principal stress
hormone, and high levels are a strong risk factor in cardiovascular
diseases and Alzheimer's disease. Physical and psychological stresses
prompt an increase in cortisol—and that begs the questions, Who
in this day and age is *not* stressed, and what impact does stress have
on the risk of Syndrome X?

Some researchers have suggested that insulin resistance and
Syndrome X are "preclinical" forms of Cushing's disease, a well-

established endocrine disease caused by the overproduction of cortisol. Cushing's disease can be caused by the excessive or chronic use of hydrocortisone, prednisone, and other steroid hormones. Because of the use of these drugs, a wide range of people, from arthritics to body builders, can be at risk for Cushing's disease.

The hormonal flux triggered by insulin can also lead to behavioral changes, which may further increase the risk of coronary heart disease. Two stress hormones—corticotropin and cortisol—are very sensitive to physical and mental stresses. Feelings of physical fatigue, mental exhaustion, and anger are strongly associated with unbalanced levels of these hormones—and with Syndrome X, as well.

Insulin, Aging, and Cancer

Incredibly, insulin has still more biological effects. It is one of the most ancient hormones in living creatures, and its hormonal antecedents can be found in insects and mollusks. As a powerful *mitogen,* insulin stimulates the division (mitogenesis) of cells and the activation of genes. Prolonged exposure to high levels of insulin actually changes the genetic behavior of cells, making them act more like older (instead of younger) cells.

Many scientists believe that every cell in the body is programmed to divide a finite number of times before its descendants die out. By accelerating cell division, insulin speeds up this process, leading to the creation of biologically older cells in a relatively young or middle-aged body.

There is also substantial evidence that elevated levels of insulin increase the risk of colon, liver, pancreatic, breast, and endometrial cancer. Insulin has been shown, in animal studies, to promote the growth of precancerous colon lesions, which often turn into cancers. Other experiments have found that insulin injections increase the growth of similar lesions. Diabetic individuals have an increased risk of developing at least some cancers, strongly suggesting that insulin resistance plays a part in tumor growth.

According to an article in the *Journal of the National Cancer Institute,* insulin itself may play a principal role in cancer growth. Conversely, the control of insulin and glucose levels may limit tumor growth. John T. A. Ely of the University of Washington, Seattle, has pointed out that insulin resistance is common in cancer patients. In contrast, tumors do not grow, or grow poorly, in underfed—that is, calorie-restricted—animals.

Insulin and Other Diseases

Elevated insulin levels have been linked to many other diseases, including behavioral and neurological disorders. Several studies have established insulin resistance as a factor in cognitive disorders and impaired thinking processes, dementia, and even Alzheimer's disease.

Insulin also affects the levels of essential nutrients in the blood. A study of diabetic patients found that insulin injections decreased blood levels of vitamin E. The reason was not clear, though the researcher thought that insulin might have some free-radical-generating properties.

DEFICIENT NUTRIENTS: THE MISSING LINK IN SYNDROME X

The conventional explanations behind Syndrome X and diabetes focus on the effect of refined dietary sugars and other carbohydrates, as well as on individual genetic susceptibility. This line of thinking provides only a partial picture of these disorders' causes, however.

The increase in destructive free radicals released by glucose, and possibly also by insulin, points to another way that diet influences susceptibility to these disorders. Free radicals and antioxidants are essentially two sides of the same coin, and free radicals are quenched by dietary antioxidants, which include vitamins E and C and alpha lipoic acid.

Antioxidant vitamins, other types of vitamins, minerals, and other micronutrients are routinely stripped away through extensive food processing and refining. As a consequence, many people live with low-grade vitamin and mineral deficiencies that limit their ability to properly manage glucose and insulin.

What nearly every researcher and writer on the subject of Syndrome X and diabetes has missed is this: *The modern diet high in sugars and other refined carbohydrates is also virtually devoid of antioxidant vitamins, other types of vitamins, minerals, and other micronutrients.* These nutrients play pivotal roles in properly metabolizing *all* carbohydrates, and the same food-processing brush stroke that increases the amount of refined carbohydrates also removes crucial vitamins and minerals. Restoring these micronutrients can play a major role in controlling glucose and insulin levels and in slowing and reversing glucose- and insulin-dependent disease processes. Indeed, many studies have shown that the addition of these nutrients can often normalize glucose function in diabetics.

For many years, medical researchers assumed that free radicals existed, but only so briefly that they could not cause any damage. In the late 1940s and early 1950s, physician and researcher Denham Harman was thinking about a universal cause of aging. He assumed that because all living creatures age and die, there had to be a common underlying cause. In 1954, he conceived the "free radical theory of aging."

Today, researchers recognize that virtually every disease process is caused or exacerbated by free radicals. They are present in heart disease, cancer, and Alzheimer's disease. Any disease that involves inflammation, from infection to rheumatoid arthritis, is free-radical dependent because inflammation generates free radicals and is itself maintained by the presence of free radicals. Even dental disorders, such as gingivitis and temporomandibular joint (TMJ) disease, involve free radicals.

Because diabetics age at a faster rate than nondiabetics, it was no surprise for scientists to discover that they routinely suffer from a heavy burden of free radicals in their bodies. Diabetics also tend to be shortchanged when it comes to antioxidants. In diabetics and people with Syndrome X, many of these free radicals are generated by high blood levels of glucose.

A team of British researchers recently compared levels of free radicals and antioxidants among insulin-dependent diabetics, non-insulin-dependent diabetics, and healthy subjects. The insulin-dependent diabetics (that is, people injecting themselves with insulin) had the lowest levels of antioxidants, perhaps because of oxidative stress induced by high glucose and by insulin injections. The non-insulin-dependent diabetics fared better, but neither group of diabetics could match the antioxidant levels of healthy subjects. Vitamins E and C provided the lion's share of the subjects' antioxidants. Another study found higher levels of "lipid peroxides," an indicator of free-radical damage in both insulin-dependent and non-insulin-dependent diabetics, compared with healthy subjects.

Not surprisingly, the levels of antioxidants in diabetics predict their susceptibility to disease. This is true of nearly every disease process, and people who consume the largest quantities of antioxidants (through vegetables and supplements) tend to have the lowest risk of developing nearly all diseases.

While Syndrome X, diabetes, and many other diseases are triggered by diets high in refined carbohydrates, there is another part of the picture that researchers have largely overlooked. The same diet that results in abnormally high glucose and insulin levels also lacks the antioxidants and other micronutrients that would help the body manage those carbohydrates.

The implications are significant. Any attempt to control Syndrome X—and disease in general—must (1) correct the basic diet and (2) use specific nutritional supplements to further reduce the risk of disease. In the next chapter, we explore the origins of nutritional medicine, its rationale and some of the evidence supporting it, and the resistance to it. We also discuss why nutritional therapy is inherently safer and more effective than drug therapy.

CHAPTER 5

The Case for Nutritional Therapies over Drugs

WOULDN'T IT BE EASY if your doctor could simply write you a prescription for a drug to improve how your body handles glucose, to burn off your extra weight, to lower your cholesterol, and to reduce your blood pressure? Many people try to follow this exact approach—and end up taking four or more drugs and then dealing with an array of unwanted side effects. We do *not* believe drug therapy is the best approach for correcting Syndrome X, though it does have its place and can sometimes complement nutritional therapies.

The reason for our belief is that nutrients and drugs work in very different ways. Nutrients are naturally occurring substances with essential roles in the human body. They are necessary for health and for life itself. Without adequate levels of nutrients, people become sick. Eating a wholesome diet and taking supplemental nutrients, such as vitamins, can help promote normal biochemical processes in the body.

In contrast, drugs are synthetic substances that play no essential roles in health. While some prescription drugs may be helpful in treating Syndrome X, it is important to remember that this disorder does not result from a lack of prescription drugs, and that prescription drugs should not be its sole treatment.

Pharmaceutical medicine began rising to prominence in the nineteenth century, when medicine was searching for a "magic bullet" capable of destroying disease-causing bacteria without harming the body. It was born of the idea that humans can alter and control nature with interventions they devise themselves. This idea is terribly misguided, however. Prescription drugs cause tens of thousands of deaths and millions of dangerous adverse reactions each year. They tamper with our biological nature and too often make things worse, not better.

THE DANGERS OF PHARMACEUTICAL DRUGS

With annual U.S. revenues of about $100 billion and worldwide revenues of $300 billion, the pharmaceutical industry is one of the largest, most powerful industries, producing some of the most sophisticated marketing and advertising anywhere. Marketing is the economic equivalent to waging war—sizing up your own forces, your enemy's (the competition), and emphasizing your own strengths and your enemy's weaknesses. Marketing strategy meetings are akin to war rooms where generals map out their plans for attack and defense.

With what seem to be almost limitless financial resources, pharmaceutical companies help shape much of a physician's education during medical school. After school, drug companies become the principal influence on physician thinking through seminars, visits from drug salespeople, and even social gatherings. The message doctors hear is that one drug is better than another, and all drugs are better than vitamins, minerals, and herbs.

Ideally, physicians should be immune to such sales pressures, but they are only human. The pressures of running a medical practice limit the time for independently checking out research. The vision of doctors becomes obscured, and under intense pressure—including the pressure to do something for their patients—they usually write a prescription.

The reality is that drugs are very toxic substances. Nutrition researcher Bernard Rimland, of San Diego, describes pharmaceutical medicine as the practice of giving patients "sublethal doses of toxic substances." Rimland has pointed out that the *Physicians' Desk Reference,* the leading compendium of drug information for doctors, consists mostly of warnings, side effects, and contraindications. Take all the scary stuff out of the 3,000-page book, Rimland says, and you'll be left with only about 150 pages describing the benefits of drugs. You can do this calculation yourself—virtually every public library has a copy of the *Physicians' Desk Reference* in its collection.

One 1990s study, published in the journal *Lancet,* found that the number of deaths from prescription drug medication errors tripled between 1983 and 1993 in the United States, while other types of fatal poisonings and population size remained fairly constant.

Another study, published in *JAMA* (*Journal of the American Medical Association*), investigated the number of adverse drug reactions over a typical year. The researchers calculated that 106,000 hospitalized patients die annually because of adverse drug reactions and that 2,216,000 other hospitalized patients have serious but nonfatal drug reactions. Given these numbers, the researchers pointed out that adverse drug reactions could rank as the fourth leading cause of death, after heart disease, cancer, and stroke. (The researchers did not address the issue of adverse drug reactions and deaths among nonhospitalized patients, so the total numbers are probably far higher.) Shocking as it may sound, legally prescribed drugs kill more people than illegal street drugs!

When this study was published in 1998, a shock wave rippled through the field of medicine. Some physicians responded by saying that there is always a benefits/risk ratio with prescription drugs, and that the benefits outweigh the risks. Rimland framed the issue a little differently. He said the drug deaths were comparable to a jumbo jet crashing and killing its passengers every day of the year. If passenger jets crashed that often, the federal government would shut down the airline industry. When it comes to deaths caused by drugs, however, the Food and Drug Administration (FDA) too often makes a habit of looking the other way.

James A. Duke, a U.S. Department of Agriculture (USDA) medical botanist and author of *The Green Pharmacy,* has pointed out that adverse drug reactions cost U.S. residents more than $136 billion annually—an amount greater than the $100 billion revenues earned by the drug companies. In other words, prescription drugs cost our society more than the economic benefits reaped by the industry. Undoubtedly, adverse drug reactions are a serious problem in other countries, though the scale of the problem has not been documented as carefully.

In contrast, the modest use of safe vitamin supplements would greatly reduce hospitalization costs. Pracon Inc., a hospital-outcomes analysis firm in Reston, Virginia, has estimated that U.S. health-care expenses could be reduced by $7.7 billion annually if consumers simply took vitamin E supplements. In another study, researchers calculated that supplements of folic acid, a zinc-containing multivitamin, and vitamin E could cut hospitalization costs by $20 billion by reducing the risk of birth defects, low-weight premature births, and coronary heart disease.

If you consider that 45 percent of North Americans—practically half of the population—have at least one chronic disease, there are incredible opportunities to use nutritional supplements and more general dietary improvements (instead of drugs) to improve health and reduce health-care costs.

The Problems with Drugs for Insulin Resistance

More specifically, there are serious problems with drugs designed to treat insulin resistance, diabetes, and the individual conditions associated with Syndrome X. The fundamental problems are that (1) drugs cannot correct nutritional deficiencies or imbalances; (2) drugs that lower cholesterol or hypertension have no effect on the underlying insulin resistance of Syndrome X; (3) many drugs actually interfere with how the body uses nutrients, exacerbating deficiencies and imbalances; and (4) many drugs increase the risk of other diseases. Some specific examples follow:

CHOLESTEROL-LOWERING DRUGS. *Statins* are one of the most popular classes of cholesterol-lowering drugs: They inhibit the body's production of cholesterol, but they do so at a point that also blocks the body's production of other important compounds. One of these compounds is coenzyme Q_{10} (CoQ_{10}), a vitamin-like substance that cells need to produce energy. A lack of CoQ_{10} appears to be a primary cause of heart failure. The irony is that taking a statin drug to lower cholesterol thereby increases the likelihood of heart failure. There is also evidence that CoQ_{10} protects against cancer and that statins may therefore increase the risk of cancer. Statins also interfere with the body's production of *squalene,* another compound that may protect against cancer.

BLOOD-PRESSURE-LOWERING DRUGS. *Calcium-channel blockers* are one of the most common types of drugs used to treat hypertension. They have also been linked to higher rates of cancer. According to a study published in *Lancet,* using calcium-channel blockers for 5 years will add 8 new cancers over 5 years and 16 new cancers over 10 years per 100 people. Is a drug worth a 16 percent increase in the risk of cancer? While such drugs are very effective in lowering blood pressure, they do not have any effect on insulin resistance or elevated insulin levels, which are the underlying cause of most types of hypertension. Calcium-channel blockers merely treat a symptom, while allowing the underlying disease process to continue.

WEIGHT-LOSS DRUGS. It seems that anyone with a few pounds to shed would love to take a "fat-burning" pill and watch fat evaporate while eating snack foods in front of the TV. It's wishful thinking. No single pill will burn off pounds.

The most recent disaster with weight-loss drugs involved Redux (fenfluramine), which was designed to reduce appetite by altering levels of neurotransmitters in the brain. Many physicians prescribed both fenfluramine and phentermine, another weight-loss drug, in a combination known as fen-phen. This drug combination was very effective in helping people lose weight. It was also very effective in causing permanent damage to their heart valves. The FDA banned Redux in 1997.

Again, fenfluramine and phentermine did nothing to alter insulin resistance, the underlying cause of obesity. Losing weight requires some effort (which we discuss in coming chapters), including changes in the composition of the food being consumed, an increase in physical activity, and some well-chosen supplements. A silver-bullet drug that sounds too good to be true probably is too good to be true.

DIABETES/INSULIN-RESISTANCE DRUGS. Adult-onset diabetes has traditionally been treated with a combination of hypoglycemic drugs (to lower blood-sugar levels) and a diet to reduce obesity associated with diabetes. Since the early 1990s, drug companies have marketed several new drugs that improve insulin sensitivity and reduce triglycerides. Not surprisingly, these drugs are being prescribed increasingly for insulin resistance and prediabetes. They are not, however, without undesirable consequences.

Rezulin (troglitazone) was approved by the FDA early in 1997 for the treatment of a limited number of diabetics. Later that year, the FDA permitted the drug to be used in the treatment of any adult-onset diabetic. Troglitazone can dramatically reduce glucose levels and decrease insulin resistance. However, several months after it was introduced, researchers noted that it increased the risk of severe liver disease. As a consequence, the drug's European distributor voluntarily halted sales of troglitazone. More recently, a study by Japanese researchers found that troglitazone actually increased hunger in diabetics taking the drug, which would probably promote overeating and obesity. Troglitazone is still being prescribed in the United States.

Glucophage (metformin hydrochloride) is another popular antidiabetes drug increasingly being used to reduce insulin resistance (improve insulin sensitivity). If the purpose of such a drug is to reduce symptoms of diabetes and the risk of heart disease, the warning on its package insert is disturbing: "The administration of oral antidiabetic drugs has been reported to be associated with increased cardiovascular mortality as compared to treatment with diet alone or diet plus insulin." In other words, metformin may improve some indicators of diabetes, but it will be more likely to cause a fatal heart attack than other therapies.

There is also unequivocal evidence that metformin substantially reduces blood levels of folic acid and vitamin B_{12} and increases levels of homocysteine. These changes are significant because folic acid (a B vitamin) and vitamin B_{12} help maintain normal DNA, and homocysteine is a protein by-product that damages the arteries and increases the risk of heart disease and stroke. Once again, using a synthetic drug to alter some aspects of insulin resistance and diabetes ratchets up the risk of other serious diseases. The "cure" throws a wrench into the body's workings, and it is as dangerous as the disease.

Perhaps the most disturbing use of metformin is as a "life-extension" drug by some alternative and self-styled "antiaging" physicians. There is a virtual cult of doctors that uses pharmaceutical drugs, as well as nutritional supplements, to slow the aging process. While many nutritional supplements are safe—and do, in fact, protect cells from many of the ravages of aging—drugs are much more unpredictable in their negative side effects. Metformin may reduce insulin resistance, but it increases the rate of cell damage and aging—hardly a reasonable trade-off.

The use of pharmaceutical drugs to treat the symptoms of diabetes and Syndrome X focuses chiefly on reducing some symptoms, but not on the underlying causes of these disorders. Nearly every drug marketed poses significant and undesirable side effects, and the social and economic costs of these drugs frequently outweigh their benefits. Given this situation, the use of pharmaceutical drugs—other than in clearly life-threatening situations—is too often irrational and dangerous.

TREATING NUTRITIONAL DISEASES NUTRITIONALLY

Syndrome X is a nutritional disease—caused primarily by the over-consumption of refined sugars and other carbohydrates. For this reason alone, it seems more rational to treat it nutritionally instead of pharmaceutically. Nutritional therapies *do* work—and they work exceptionally well. Consider the dramatic benefits of just one recent dietary study by physician Michel de Lorgeril.

Physicians and nutritionists generally believe that the traditional Mediterranean-style diet reduces the risk of heart disease, one of the principal consequences of Syndrome X. The diet is rich in simple, nutritious foods, including vegetables, fruit, fish, legumes, and olive oil. Many of these foods contain nutrients (such as antioxidants and beneficial fats) that decrease the likelihood of Syndrome X, reduce the accumulation of body fat, and lower blood fats and blood pressure. The traditional Mediterranean diet is also relatively low in refined carbohydrates, so it does not stimulate large increases in glucose and insulin.

In his study, de Lorgeril asked more than 400 men and women, all of whom had suffered a heart attack, either to switch to a Mediterranean-style diet or to continue eating their regular diets. Over the next four years, de Lorgeril found that people eating the Mediterranean-style diet had a 50–70 percent lower risk of experiencing a second heart attack, compared with the people who continued eating their original diets. This lower risk was strongly associated with improvements in total cholesterol and blood pressure, two of the components of Syndrome X.

As if these health benefits were not impressive enough, the study revealed other things, as well. The reduction in heart-disease deaths among people eating the Mediterranean diet was far superior to that achieved by cholesterol-lowering drugs in other studies. In addition, the Mediterranean diet did not cause any of the undesirable side effects common to drugs.

Furthermore, patient *compliance*—the willingness to follow doctors' instructions—over the four-year study was exceptionally high. The majority of patients stuck with the prescribed Mediterranean diet, contradicting the stereotype that diets are hard to follow and that medications are preferable because they are less of a hassle. Although de Lorgeril did not explore why patients eating the Mediterranean diet were so cooperative, it may have been simply because the foods tasted better than what the patients had been eating previously.

Like dietary studies, investigations and clinical experiences with micronutrient supplements (described in later chapters) have also resulted in tremendous health benefits. Various supplements, such as alpha lipoic acid, vitamin E, chromium, and silymarin (an herbal extract) can have dramatic effects on glucose levels, Syndrome X, diabetes, and heart disease. Consider that a British study of 2,000 men and women found that supplements of natural vitamin E—a nutrient removed when grains are refined—reduced the risk of heart disease by 77 percent.

The Nutrition Rationale

In an era that focuses increasingly on gene research and gene therapy, it has become too easy to forget the fundamental importance of nutrition. All life depends on a steady supply of high-quality nutrients, and human beings are no exception to this rule. Although our genes contain the biological instructions for life and influence the risk of many diseases, they depend on nutrients to function normally. Nutrients form the most basic chemical building blocks of our bodies and minds, down to the level of molecules and atoms.

Unfortunately, because of extensive food processing and refining, much of the modern diet provides a lopsided serving of nutrients with far too many refined carbohydrates, seriously unbalanced fats, and inadequate levels of most vitamins and minerals. This unbalanced diet (discussed more in the next chapter) has undermined our health and our resistance to disease. The consequences include the growing prevalence of Syndrome X and its associated health problems.

Despite the fundamental role nutrition plays in health, many physicians remain skeptical about nutritional therapies and vitamin supplements, believing there is only limited research to support their use. It turns out that a vast amount of research has been conducted on dietary therapies and vitamins, minerals, and other supplements.

These nutrition and supplement studies include human trials, epidemiological studies, animal experiments, and cell-culture studies. In weighing the totality of the research, it becomes very clear that simple, traditional diets and high levels of vitamins and minerals are almost always associated with optimal biological performance and good health. In contrast, highly refined modern diets and low levels of vitamins and minerals are almost always associated with poor biological health and disease.

We offer a few supporting numbers, which may surprise you, to convey the volume of research. In 1998 alone, more than 1,000 studies on vitamin E and almost 700 studies on vitamin C were published in medical and other scientific journals. Most of these studies showed positive relationships between nutrition and health. In 1998, also, more than 5,500 studies were published on vitamins per se and more than 3,200 studies were published on antioxidants. Since the Medline database was started in 1966, more than 147,000 studies on vitamins have been published. More than one third of these articles—50,000—were published between 1990 and 1998. More research—most of it positive—has been published on nutrients than on most drugs! The problem is not a dearth of vitamin research; it is the task of keeping up with all the research.

The Need for Better Nutrition

Although we explore problems with the modern diet in the next chapter, it is important to make several important points before going any further. One, everything that we are, as biological creatures, depends on the nutrients we consume. Nutrients provide the raw materials for the physical structure of our bodies (including our minds), and these raw materials are converted to thousands of biochemicals needed for us to grow, heal, and function normally. Nutrition may even be more important than genetics because some studies have found that genetic diseases (e.g., Down syndrome and mitochondrial myopathies) can be improved through diet and supplements.

Two, many dietitians and physicians recommend that people consume "balanced" diets to maintain health, as if this were the beginning and end of all things nutritional. Unfortunately, the concept of a balanced diet is often in the eyes of the beholder, and people eating poor diets often believe they are receiving balanced nutrition. Furthermore, the concept of a balanced diet has been unduly influenced by the major food industries producing and selling meat, dairy products, and grains.

Three, the notion that people can easily obtain and consume a balanced, or nutritious, diet is based largely on unfounded assumptions. In truth, eating well is easier said than done when you consider that entire aisles of supermarkets are devoted to tempting soft drinks ("liquid candy"), sugar-laden breakfast cereals, and cookies and candies. Many people do not understand the nuances of food labels, which meet the letter of the law but ignore the fact that the average person is not a chemist or a food-and-drug lawyer. For example, how many consumers understand the difference between "orange juice" and "orange juice drink"? (The latter contains only about 10 percent orange juice.) Inundated with thousands of manufactured foods of dubious nutritional value, it becomes difficult to navigate the aisles of supermarkets. It should also be no surprise, given the preponderance of refined carbohydrates in these aisles, that Syndrome X is rampant.

In so many ways, nutrition has become the "missing link" in modern medicine. Although it has a fundamental influence on our health, it has also been routinely ignored and undervalued for many years.

In the next chapter, we describe how our diet has gone wrong, particularly during the industrialization of our food supply and what has become the "fast-food era." Our reference point is the diet of the past, the foods that human beings evolved eating. Then, in subsequent chapters, we turn these concepts into highly practical advice. We explain a number of dietary principles to help guide you safely and nutritiously through the modern food supply. We also offer some menu plans and recipes with the hope of awakening your taste buds to the wonderful flavors of wholesome foods. You will discover that good food can be tasty—and that it can protect you from Syndrome X.

CHAPTER 6

The Diet We Were Made For and How It Changed

MOST OF US don't think much about the food we eat. The fact of the matter is that we have strayed a long way from the food we were meant to eat. This is exactly what has gotten us into trouble with Syndrome X—and with many other modern diseases, for that matter.

In this chapter, we describe what our distant ancestors ate, and then we take you on a quick trip down food history lane. By understanding the kinds of foods humans evolved on—and then learning how human diets significantly changed with the agricultural, industrial, and fast-food revolutions—you will gain a much clearer picture of why Syndrome X has emerged as a widespread, modern disease.

As we mentioned, we begin by explaining the diet of our Stone Age, or Paleolithic, ancestors, who lived 15,000 to 40,000 years ago. By understanding the past, we have a starting point by which to understand our basic dietary requirements. From that starting point, we can gain a sense of direction for the present and the future. It is important to remember that human beings coevolved with their foods. In other words, we all grew up together, in effect, on the same street on Earth, and we are genetically dependent on the nutrients in simple, whole foods.

If you don't believe in evolution, please refrain from dismissing our line of thinking too quickly. Consider what we write in a slightly different way: that we are not eating the wholesome foods God intended us to eat, and the resulting dietary discrepancy between past and present undermines our health.

AN OVERVIEW OF THE PALEOLITHIC DIET

Although most people don't think about it in this way, early humans were the original health-food nuts, subsisting entirely on fresh, organic foods. Paleolithic people, of course, were hunter-gatherers: they sustained themselves by hunting large and small animals, catching fish and shellfish, and gathering edible plants. They rarely ate grains (and no cultivated grains), and they never consumed dairy products (other than mother's milk during infancy), domesticated meats, pressed oils or fats, refined carbohydrates, or alcohol. They also never ate refined sugars (other than occasionally honey, which was troublesome to obtain!).

Paleolithic people ate an incredibly diverse diet that supplied vitamins and minerals far in excess of the standard levels officially recommended today, such as the Recommended Dietary Allowances (RDAs) or Reference Daily Intakes (RDIs). S. Boyd Eaton, a medical expert on the Paleolithic diet, has estimated that the average Paleolithic diet included more than 200 different species of plants—perhaps 10 to 40 times more variety than in the diet typically eaten by people in modern countries, such as the United States, Canada, and Britain. Paleolithic foods were also usually eaten within hours of being obtained, with little if any alteration and often without cooking.

To give you a sense of how foods have changed, we first briefly describe the types of carbohydrates eaten by our Paleolithic ancestors and then how carbohydrates have changed since that time. Afterward, we take a similar, quick look at protein, fats, and micronutrients (vitamins and minerals). By looking at these specific categories of nutrients, you will see how the diet we were biologically designed for has declined and how modern processed foods have set the stage for Syndrome X.

CARBOHYDRATES PAST AND PRESENT

Carbohydrates, consisting of starches and sugars, are the body's principal "energy food." During digestion, the body breaks carbohydrates down into glucose, which cells burn (or oxidize) to create energy. The process is analogous to burning a log or a piece of coal for energy.

There are two main groups of carbohydrates: *refined carbohydrates,* including bread, snack foods, and various forms of sugar, which are digested very quickly and lead to rapid increases in glucose and insulin, and *complex carbohydrates,* which contain complex sugars and starches and various types of fiber, all of which are digested slowly and moderate the glucose and insulin response. Complex carbohydrates are found in vegetables, beans and other legumes, and some types of fruit (e.g., berries and apples).

Carbohydrates in the Paleolithic Diet

Paleolithic humans obtained about half of their daily energy (caloric) intake from carbohydrates, roughly the same percentage generally recommended today. However, Paleolithic carbohydrates differed greatly from those that most people now eat.

The bulk of carbohydrates in the Paleolithic diet came from uncultivated vegetables, which were obtained by foraging. According to C. Leigh Broadhurst, a visiting scientist at the USDA in Beltsville, Maryland, these plants bore little resemblance to the highly cultivated fruits and vegetables most people consume today. Many of the Paleolithic vegetables tended to resemble kale, a vegetable whose modern descendant remains unappetizing to most people.

In addition, fruit was not a major dietary staple; it was not eaten at all in the northern latitudes, and not in the winter in temperate zones. The fruits that did exist were small and wild—often resembling wild rose hips. They did not resemble today's sweet, succulent fruits with their high sugar content.

The plant foods eaten by our Stone Age ancestors were also bulkier and had much more fiber than modern foods. The Paleolithic diet provided more than 100 grams of fiber daily, compared with less than 20 grams daily in today's diet.

High-fiber foods have a number of beneficial effects. They require more chewing and thus slower eating, and they create a feeling of fullness; an equivalent sense of fullness can be obtained only by eating larger amounts of modern refined foods. In terms of preventing Syndrome X, fiber limits the digestibility of plant starches and helps buffer natural sugars, thus avoiding sharp increases in glucose and insulin. In general, uncultivated plant foods—the kinds that were eaten in the Paleolithic era—release glucose very slowly into the bloodstream, thus triggering only modest, gradual increases in insulin.

PALEOLITHIC VERSUS MODERN CARBOHYDRATES

Then	Now
Large number of plant foods	Limited number of plant foods
Many nutrient-rich vegetables	Relatively few vegetables
Unprocessed carbohydrates	Highly refined carbohydrates (e.g., pastas)
100 grams daily of dietary fiber	20 grams daily of dietary fiber
No cultivated grains	Large intake of cultivated grains

Paleolithic men and woman rarely ate cereal grains (such as wheat or maize), and they never ate cultivated grains. By contrast, most dietary carbohydrates today are in the form of highly refined grain products. Bread accounts for 15 percent of the carbohydrates consumed by people today; even contemporary whole-wheat bread is virtually devoid of fiber, by Paleolithic standards.

How Carbohydrates Have Changed

About 10,000 years ago—just a smidgen of time in evolutionary terms—our ancestors began eating foods higher in carbohydrates, such as whole grains and legumes. This shift from high-protein meats as a centerpiece of the diet to high-carbohydrate grains has often been described in superlative terms, such as the dawn of the Agricultural Revolution. In truth, people had little choice but to develop agriculture because of a shortage of large game animals (probably because of overhunting). Grains allowed humans to obtain the calories they needed to survive the meat shortage. However, the switch compromised health, and this effect became more serious with the refining of grains.

About 2,000 years ago, people began using grinding stones to make whole-grain flours. Before machine technology was developed during the Industrial Revolution in the 1800s, however, only royalty and the rich ate nutrient- and fiber-stripped white flour because it was very labor intensive and costly to produce. As a result, obesity and degenerative diseases such as heart disease and adult-onset diabetes—consequences of Syndrome X—often afflicted mainly the royalty and the wealthy.

As the processing of grains became technically easier and less costly, Syndrome X started to affect larger numbers of people (though, of course, the condition was not recognized until relatively recently). Perhaps the most serious decline in the diet began with the advent of the steel roller mill in the late 1800s. The steel roller mill made the refining of whole-wheat grains and sugar cane a fast and inexpensive process, and the resulting white flour and white sugar became affordable and easily available to the general population.

Although societies around the world did not exhibit immediate health problems from eating white flour and white sugar, they did slowly but surely develop them. Over time—just enough time to prevent people from readily connecting the cause with the effect—Syndrome X and diabetes began to affect more people.

A few astute researchers did notice this connection. For example, T. L. Cleave traced the development of hypertension, diabetes, and heart disease to the increased intake of refined carbohydrates. In every case Cleave studied, he found that primitive cultures were almost entirely free of these diseases until about 20 years after white sugar and white flour were introduced. This pattern was so consistent that Cleave named the phenomenon the "Rule of 20 Years." However, most scientists remained oblivious to how changes in the food supply were affecting health.

As convenience markets and supermarkets started sprouting up across the United States, more food products made out of refined carbohydrates infiltrated our diets. Food manufacturers began to realize that by polishing rice and degerminating and bleaching flour, they could make grain products so nutritionally sterile that insects could not survive eating them. White-flour-based convenience products with long shelf lives became accepted as wholesome foods, and foods such as white bread and buns became staples.

In the 1930s, health professionals noticed that people who ate white bread suffered from health problems caused by deficiencies of vitamins B_1, B_2, B_3, and iron. The government responded by passing the Enrichment Act of 1942, which required manufacturers to enrich white flour with these four nutrients. However, white flour was and still is missing at least 20 other nutrients.

Similarly, white sugar, a highly refined product from nutrient- and fiber-rich sugar cane, provides nothing except empty calories: It's void of fiber, vitamins, and minerals. Sugar was a rare treat in the infancy of this country. Now, each year excessive sugar intake displaces an average of 150 pounds of other, more nutritious foods in people's diets.

Both white flour and sugar lack chromium, magnesium, and zinc—all essential minerals that help the body properly use carbohydrates. Without adequate levels of these minerals (which you will read about in Chapter 14), insulin resistance and Syndrome X develop at an accelerated pace.

White flour and sugar may be the worst contributors to these conditions, but there is still more to the story. The more industrialized and convenience-oriented our society has become, the more processed carbohydrates have become—and *the more processed carbohydrates become, the more they increase blood sugar and insulin levels.* For example, canned vegetables and beans, which started to become popular in the 1950s, raise blood sugar and insulin more than their fresh counterparts do. Similarly, highly concentrated fruit juices raise blood sugar and insulin more than fresh, fiber-rich fruit.

Since the Paleolithic era, carbohydrates have become increasingly carbohydrate dense—in other words, these foods now have more grams of carbohydrates per serving and have become much lower in blood-sugar-regulating nutrients and fiber. These changes in dietary carbohydrates account in large part for the increasing prevalence of Syndrome X. In addition, dramatic changes in protein intake also contributed to the rise of this condition.

PROTEIN PAST AND PRESENT

During digestion, protein is broken down into amino acids, which are re-formed into proteins the body needs for various functions. Protein makes up much of the physical structure of the body, including skin, nails, organs, and glands. Proteins are also the building blocks of enzymes and many of the body's hormones.

The body can convert some protein to energy, but it is digested slowly and therefore stabilizes glucose and insulin levels.

Protein in the Paleolithic Diet

The amount of protein eaten by our distant ancestors varied with the season and geographic location, but the average amount consumed was about 35 percent of the total diet—almost three times what the average person eats today. Much of the protein consumed during Paleolithic times came from what we now call game meat— wild animals that were hunted, not bred. Because wild animals moved about freely (in contrast to animals kept in a pen), their meat was higher in protein (muscle) and significantly lower in total fat and saturated fat than most commercial meats sold today.

PROTEIN AND FAT CONTENT OF MEAT

Wild game meat (e.g., venison, rabbit, and buffalo) is similar in composition to the meat people ate in Paleolithic times. Compared with domestic meat (e.g., beef and pork), wild game meat is higher in protein and lower in fat, which makes it a healthier food. On average, wild game meat contains approximately 22 grams of protein per 100-gram portion, whereas domestic meat contains only about 16 grams of protein. Wild game meat also contains an average of only 4 grams of fat in a 100-gram portion, compared with 29 grams of fat in domesticated meat.

Another way of looking at the protein/fat issue: Common supermarket meat (including hamburger, sirloin, and pork loin) contains more than six times the amount of fat and only about three fourths the amount of protein found in game meat. People did not evolve eating meat with substantially more fat than protein.

The meat found in the Paleolithic diet had other beneficial properties, as well. It was rich in omega-3 fats (often called "fatty acids"), a family of healthy dietary fats that helps prevent insulin resistance, Syndrome X, and heart disease. (You'll find out more about the health benefits of omega-3 fatty acids in the next chapter.) There is also considerable evidence that the earliest humans evolved in the Rift Valley of eastern Africa, where they consumed large amounts of lake fish and shellfish, which are particularly high in omega-3 fatty acids.

How Protein Has Changed

When our ancestors began eating more grains, their protein intake decreased, and this in turn resulted in health problems rarely seen before—such as tooth decay, bone malformations, and heart disease. There is evidence that, in ancient Egypt, a high-carbohydrate, low-protein diet (similar to the high-carbohydrate Food Pyramid diet recommended today) led to the early onset of cardiovascular disease, a common complication of Syndrome X.

Despite the shift to more cultivated plant foods, most societies continued to place tremendous importance on eating animal foods for health. In North America at the beginning of the twentieth century, when degenerative diseases such as diabetes and cardiovascular disease were rare, about 30 percent of the calories in the average diet came from meat, dairy products, and eggs. At that time, more than half the population lived on farms and raised beef cattle without chemicals and hormones; kept chickens, pigs, and dairy animals at pasture; fished in creeks, rivers, lakes, and oceans; and hunted for wild game. The protein composition of the diet at the turn of the century was not significantly different from that found in the diet of Paleolithic people, except that the meat was not quite as lean, and dairy products were consumed.

Just as dietary carbohydrates changed for the worse throughout the twentieth century, so did dietary protein. Ranchers began to fatten up animals on such foods as corn and soybeans (high in carbohydrates and omega-6 fatty acids) instead of letting them eat their natural diet of grass (rich in omega-3 fatty acids). The combination of a grain-based diet and lack of exercise (because animals were penned up) fattened up these animals, and it drastically altered the protein and fatty-acid profile of meat.

Other changes occurred, as well. Fish consumption declined, and as more and more people began to eat domesticated beef and dairy products, antibiotics and hormones were added to livestock feed to increase meat production. In addition, pesticides and pollutants from the environment ended up in meat on the dinner table. Later, as fast foods and convenience foods increased in number, food manufacturers began adding more preservatives and additives, including sugar, salt, and sodium-based preservatives, to make processed meat products that had longer shelf lives. Ready-to-eat meat products became more available to the masses, but they were nutritionally inferior to the type of animal protein our distant ancestors thrived on.

Although the changes that occurred with carbohydrates have had a more direct effect on the development of Syndrome X, the changes in protein foods have also adversely affected health and indirectly contributed to the development of insulin resistance. This is especially true because today's animal protein is derived from animals fed a high-grain diet. You will learn more about this in the next chapter when we discuss how to correct the diet to prevent and reverse Syndrome X.

FATS PAST AND PRESENT

With all the bad news about fats, it's easy to forget that these are essential nutrients. Like carbohydrates, they are a ready energy source for the body. Unlike carbohydrates, fats have many other beneficial functions.

Fats form much of the structure of the body, from cell membranes to a biological cushion that protects us against injury. Fats also serve as insulation, preventing the loss of body heat, and they also are the building blocks of important hormonelike substances known as eicosanoids and cytokines.

Fats in the Paleolithic Diet

Paleolithic people received between 20 and 25 percent of their calories as fat, and the fat came entirely from whole foods—namely, muscle meats and organ meats from wild game, nuts and seeds, and vegetables. They did not consume pressed or refined oils (e.g., corn, soy, or safflower oils) of any kind.

Some of the fat our very distant ancestors ate was saturated fat, but they also had a good balance of other dietary fats, particularly those from the omega-3, omega-6, and omega-9 families of fatty acids. Perhaps most important, Paleolithic people consumed the essential fats needed for health—omega-6 and omega-3 fatty acids—in a 1:1 to 4:1 balance. (In other words, these fats were found in relatively equal amounts in their diet.) This is the balance that humans evolved on and that supported health. This balance has become totally skewed in the modern diet, contributing to the rise in Syndrome X.

How Fats Have Changed

After the Agricultural Revolution 10,000 years ago, people began using dairy products and fats that were easily extracted from other foods. The types of dietary fats consumed since that time have included fish and fish liver oils, butter and other animal fats, flaxseed oil, sesame oil, peanut oil, olive oil, and coconut and palm oils. Although these fats differed in terms of the amounts of polyunsaturated fatty acids, monounsaturated fatty acids, and saturated fatty acids they contained, historical evidence shows that people generally remained healthy when they consumed the natural fats native to their region—as long as they also consumed a diet rich in whole foods and antioxidant nutrients (which protect fats from breaking down and becoming harmful).

After the Industrial Revolution, several events changed the nature of dietary fats, making them nutrients that degraded instead of improved health:

- Technologies were developed to use high pressures and temperatures to extract oils from corn, soy, and safflower—foods that previously had not been used as concentrated sources of fat. These refined food products are high in omega-6 fatty acids, which increased the ratio of omega-6 to omega-3 fatty acids in the diet. This abnormal ratio disrupts normal body processes and ultimately increases the risk of Syndrome X.

■ In the early 1900s, manufacturers learned how to hydrogenate oils—that is, artificially saturate liquid vegetable oils with hydrogen to form solid fats loaded with unhealthy trans-fatty acids, which increase the risk of heart disease. (You will learn more about trans-fatty acids in the next chapter.) Crisco vegetable shortening, a cheap replacement for butter made out of partially hydrogenated oil, went on sale in 1911, and other shortenings and margarines made out of partially hydrogenated oils followed.

■ In the 1930s, manufacturers began using toxic solvents to extract even more oil from plants. This brought down the cost of vegetable oils and made them available to the masses. However, the combined processes of heating vegetable oils at high temperatures, treating them with solvents, and bleaching and deodorizing them created hazardous free radicals and destroyed protective antioxidant nutrients in the oils. Refined vegetable oils, therefore, became even more unhealthy. Like white flour and sugar, these refined fats supplied calories but no nutrients beneficial to health.

During the 1960s and 1970s, many people mistakenly thought saturated fat was the chief villain in heart disease, and this belief launched an aggressive campaign against saturated fat to lower cholesterol. As saturated-fat phobia swept across the land, officials advocated the use of omega-6-rich vegetable oils and corn-oil margarines, and food companies were quick to add omega-6-rich oils and partially hydrogenated oils to all kinds of convenience food products (because they are more resistant to spoilage than omega-3 fatty acids).

The skyrocketing use of products with omega-6 fats was unfortunate because the composition of our diet therefore strayed even further from the diet our bodies were designed for. Instead of the 4:1 to 1:1 omega-6-to-omega-3 fatty-acid ratio our bodies need to thrive, the overall ratio of omega-6 to omega-3 fatty acids in the diet today is now in the range of 20:1 to 30:1. This abnormal ratio ultimately helps promote insulin resistance, Syndrome X, and heart disease.

MICRONUTRIENTS PAST AND PRESENT

Micronutrients include vitamins, minerals, and phytonutrients (such as flavonoids and carotenoids). People require relatively large quantities of carbohydrates, protein, and fats; hence, these nutrients are commonly referred to as "macronutrients." In contrast, people need much smaller quantities of vitamins, minerals, and related nutrients; that's why these nutrients are called "micronutrients."

Vitamins, minerals, and other micronutrients have extraordinarily diverse functions in health. They stimulate and regulate much of the biochemical activity that normally occurs in the body, including growth and healing. Without certain micronutrients, the body would not be able to burn carbohydrates, proteins, or fats for energy—or use them as construction materials.

Micronutrients in the Paleolithic Diet

The Paleolithic diet provided far higher levels of vitamins, minerals, and phytonutrients, compared with the modern refined diet. There are several reasons for this difference. First, Paleolithic humans consumed a large quantity of plant foods, and such foods are typically very high in most micronutrients (such as vitamins and minerals). Second, the game meats they ate also contained higher quantities of vitamins and minerals relative to their protein content. In other words, these foods were extremely nutrient dense, whereas refined carbohydrates are not. Third, Paleolithic men and women were very active physically—they had no cars or labor-saving devices, and gathering and hunting foods required physical exertion. This activity increased appetite and food consumption, which in turn increased vitamin and mineral intake.

Overall, the Paleolithic diet provided about three to five times more vitamins than those listed in the RDAs. The estimated Paleolithic intake of vitamin B_1 is 5 mg, compared to an RDA range of 1.3–1.7 mg. Paleolithic intake of vitamin C was about 439 mg daily, compared with an RDA of 60 mg and an estimated current intake of 77–109 mg daily. Likewise, Paleolithic intake of vitamin E was 28 international units (IU), compared with an RDA of 15 IU and current intake of 7–10 IU daily. Paleolithic intake of zinc was about 43 mg daily, roughly three times higher than today's intake and the RDA level. Eaton has observed that Paleolithic intake of some vitamins, such as folic acid, was so high that people would have no choice but to take supplements to achieve the same levels today.

Although vitamins and minerals are of extraordinary importance, most of the antioxidants and micronutrients in plant foods are actually *phytonutrients*—a broad class of compounds consisting chiefly of flavonoids and carotenoids (which are discussed in more detail in Chapter 15). Researchers have identified 5,000 flavonoids and 600 carotenoids, and while they do not all occur in edible plants, large numbers of them do. Studies have estimated modern flavonoid consumption to be between 23 and 170 mg daily, but 1,000 mg daily may have been more typical of Paleolithic diets. Comparisons of kale (one of the few modern foods that resembles a Paleolithic vegetable) with lettuce, cucumbers, and celery suggest that people used to consume somewhere between 5 to 24 times more phytonutrients.

How Micronutrients Have Changed

Just as carbohydrates, protein, and fats in the diet have declined, so too have the levels of virtually every micronutrient. This has occurred for several reasons. First, modern agricultural practices have severely depleted the levels of most minerals in our soil. This depletion lowers the levels of minerals in plants that grow in the soil, in animals that eat the plants, and, ultimately, in the foods people eat.

Modern shipping and distribution techniques and food processing practices have also caused nutrient levels to drop. For example, distributors nowadays pick a piece of fruit before it is ripe, then they box and ship it across the country to a supermarket. Such fruit is dramatically lower in vitamins and minerals than fruit or vegetables picked fresh off a vine or tree.

Food processing and preserving techniques have also resulted in a loss of many nutrients. Significantly, processing has reversed the dietary potassium-to-sodium ratio our bodies were designed for. Potassium is lost during food processing, and food manufacturers routinely add salt (sodium chloride) and sodium-rich preservatives to food. So, as the same food goes through processing steps, its potassium-to-sodium ratio falls dramatically.

Since the 1950s or so, as people have increasingly eaten more and more processed convenience foods, their all-important potassium-to-sodium ratio has been disrupted further. The typical adult now consumes about 25 percent more sodium than potassium, roughly 4,000 mg of sodium, compared with about 3,000 mg of potassium. This ratio is an extreme reversal of what Paleolithic folks consumed—an estimated 7,000 mg of potassium and 700 mg of sodium daily. A low potassium-to-sodium ratio increases the risk of high blood pressure, coronary heart disease, and stroke, all of which are common complications of Syndrome X.

By eating more whole, natural foods (which you'll learn more about in the next several chapters), you can bring the potassium-to-sodium ratio in your diet to a level closer to the ratio people were designed for and, therefore, help prevent many components and complications of Syndrome X.

PHYSICAL ACTIVITY PAST AND PRESENT

What has physical activity got to do with diet? Physical exertion demands increased amounts of energy-producing nutrients, otherwise known as calories.

Early humans, like their primate ancestors, had to expend considerable physical effort to obtain food. They did not drive to supermarkets or simply wander into their kitchen and contemplate the inside of a refrigerator. Foraging and hunting was hard, strenuous work and required considerable physical effort. Although Paleolithic people consumed far more calories compared with modern people, we know that they were also trimmer and more muscular, based on studies of skeletal remains. Like modern athletes, they burned off most of those calories.

Industrialization during the nineteenth and early twentieth centuries reduced the need for physical exertion. Essentially, the Industrial Revolution enabled people to leverage mechanical energy instead of their own physical energy. By one estimate, the mechanization of farming in Japan reduced physical exertion by 50 percent. In England, the use of labor-saving devices between the 1950s and 1990s reduced caloric expenditure by 65 percent.

Industrialization and technology have enabled us to save labor and to prevent considerable physical wear and tear on our bodies. However, less physical activity generally leads to a high ratio of fat to muscle cells, so more glucose is stored as fat, rather than burned for energy. Reduced physical activity, especially when combined with a high-carbohydrate, high-fat diet, has contributed to the increased prevalence of insulin resistance, obesity, and Syndrome X.

HOW OUR DIET HAS CHANGED

Looking at the pace of change in the human diet, 100,000 generations of people were hunter-gatherers, 500 generations have been agriculturists, only 10 generations have lived since the start of the industrial age, and only 2 or 3 generations have existed since the advent of highly processed and artificial foods. *Our bodies are designed for the foods eaten by our Paleolithic ancestors, not for the types of convenient, processed foods most people eat today.*

The evidence strongly suggests that our genes function best on Paleolithic foods—lots of vegetables and animal protein—and not well on the refined carbohydrates that dominate modern diets. Given a highly refined diet, our bodies tend to overreact or under-react, such as with glucose and insulin levels shooting up and metabolism slowing down.

The further we, as humans, have moved away from the Paleolithic diet, the more susceptible we have become to Syndrome X and other diet-dependent diseases. In a very real sense, the best anti-Syndrome X diet is the Paleolithic diet—or at least a more modern and convenient variation of it. In the next chapter, you'll learn exactly how to change your diet so it works with your genes to prevent and reverse Syndrome X.

PART TWO

The Anti-X Diet
and Health Program

CHAPTER 7

Redefining What to Eat: The Nine Anti-X Diet Principles

IF THE BAD NEWS IS that many of the highly processed foods of the twentieth century cause Syndrome X, the good news is that you can prevent and treat this health problem by changing your diet. Food therapy has been used for thousands of years to protect against illness. In recent years, scientific research has helped us understand much more clearly why some diets cause disease and why others promote health. Syndrome X is a nutritional disease, so understanding some basic principles of eating right is crucial to maintaining and restoring your health.

Changing your diet to control Syndrome X means that you need to rethink the food you routinely eat and get back to basics. This chapter explains the principles behind our protective *Anti-X diet*—and also explains why food is often the best medicine for treating Syndrome X.

To get you on the right track, we first quickly introduce you to our Anti-X diet principles and then take a more in-depth look at each individual principle. In Chapters 8 and 9, we explain how to follow these principles as you navigate through restaurants, supermarkets, and your own kitchen.

THE ANTI-X DIET PRINCIPLES

1. Avoid refined carbohydrates, including white flour, white rice, and white sugar and other sweeteners.
2. Eat foods in as natural and fresh a state as possible.
3. Emphasize nonstarchy vegetables as your primary sources of carbohydrates.
4. Keep your intake of nutritious carbohydrate-dense foods moderate or low, depending on your health.
5. Avoid soft drinks, fruit juices, alcohol, and other highly processed drinks.
6. Eliminate omega-6-rich vegetable oils from your diet, and use cold-pressed, extra-virgin olive oil instead.
7. Enrich your diet with omega-3 fats whenever you can.
8. Steer clear of trans-fatty acids, which are found in deep-fried foods, margarine, and foods that contain partially hydrogenated oils.
9. Eat some protein at every meal and snack.

ANTI-X PRINCIPLE 1: AVOID REFINED CARBOHYDRATES

Without question, the most important Anti-X diet guideline is to avoid refined carbohydrates. We have described in great detail how the intake of refined carbohydrates—namely, white sugar and white flour—is directly linked to the development of Syndrome X and its common consequences, including diabetes and cardiovascular disease.

Although most people understand that sugar rapidly raises glucose to very high levels, fewer people understand that white flour, found in everything from bread to pretzels, does exactly the same thing. White bread, for example, has a *glycemic-index rating*—a measurement of how high glucose levels rise after particular foods are consumed—higher than that of sugar! In other words, white bread raises glucose levels higher and faster than sugar does.

That's not the only problem with white flour. Any product that contains white flour or white sugar also lacks at least some of the nutrients and fiber needed to help the body metabolize carbohydrates efficiently. The body, therefore, must draw on its own nutrient reserves to deal with foods made out of white flour and white sugar. This ultimately leads to nutrient deficiencies—such as of chromium and other nutrients—which contribute to insulin resistance. To protect yourself against Syndrome X, you should consistently avoid refined white sugar and white flour.

The same problem exists for white rice, which is regarded as a healthy food in the USDA's Food Pyramid. White rice is stripped of the nutrients and fiber found in brown rice. Although it is fortified with iron and a few B vitamins, it is still missing numerous nutrients helpful in carbohydrate metabolism. Over time, therefore, eating nutrient-poor white rice can also lead to deficiencies, which contribute to insulin resistance.

Furthermore, just like white-flour products, white rice rapidly raises glucose to high levels. So, steering clear of white rice (including rice cakes) is also essential for reducing your risk of developing insulin resistance. Basically, white rice and white flour are no better than pure sugar because the body reacts to them essentially the same way.

There are many hidden sugars in the diet—sweeteners that find themselves in all kinds of processed convenience foods. Whether the sweetener seems fairly natural, such as honey, or is highly processed sucrose or high-fructose corn syrup, it will quickly boost blood glucose to high levels. (The one exception to this rule is fructose, a highly refined sugar made from corn. Unlike other sweeteners, fructose does not cause a spike in glucose levels, but it should be avoided because it promotes insulin resistance and raises cholesterol and triglyceride levels, as we explained in Chapter 4.)

IDENTIFYING SOURCES OF REFINED CARBOHYDRATES AND SUGARS IN THE SUPERMARKET

Refined flour is found in foods that contain enriched flour, bleached flour, unbleached flour, semolina flour, wheat flour, and flour in the list of ingredients. These foods are often light in color and include the most popular foods in the American diet—pasta, pizza crust, bagels, pretzels, tortillas, muffins, and most breads and other baked goods.

Refined rice is found in foods that contain enriched rice, polished rice, rice flour, and rice in the list of ingredients. These foods are often white or pale in color unless prepared with colored seasonings or in a colored broth.

Sugar and concentrated sweeteners are found in foods that contain any of the following: barley malt, beet sugar, brown sugar, cane juice crystals, cane sugar, corn syrup, corn syrup solids, date sugar,

dextrose, diastatic malt, fructose, fruit juice and fruit-juice concentrates, glucose, glucose solids, golden sugar, golden syrup, grape
sugar, high-fructose corn syrup, honey, invert sugar, lactose, malt
syrup, maltodextrin, maltose, mannitol, maple sugar, maple syrup,
molasses, raw sugar, refiner's syrup, sorghum syrup, sucrose, sugar,
turbinado sugar, yellow sugar.

Sugar and sweeteners are found in large amounts in most
sweets and are hidden in small amounts in the vast majority of
convenience foods. The quick way to discern sweeteners on the
label is to look for the word sugar in any form, for words ending
in -ose, and for high-fructose corn syrup, cane juice, fruit-juice
concentrates, maple syrup, and honey.

The human body simply wasn't designed to handle concentrated
sweeteners. Eating a lot of them stresses the glucose-handling
mechanisms in the body and sets in motion events that lead to overproduction of insulin and to insulin resistance. Therefore, avoiding concentrated sweeteners is essential for preventing Syndrome
X. This does not mean just avoiding obvious sources of sugars, such
as soft drinks, cookies, cakes, and candies. It also means avoiding
any foods—from cold cuts to sauces—that have sweeteners added
to them. While the sugar content of many everyday foods that contain sweeteners may not seem like that big of a deal, a few grams of
sugar here and a few grams of sugar there add up and increase the
risk of insulin resistance.

How important is it to avoid refined carbohydrates—that is,
white flour, white rice, white sugar, and other sweeteners? Very
important. A 1997 study found that women who eat large amounts
of refined carbohydrates have double the risk of developing diabetes, compared with those who eat less refined foods.

ANTI-X PRINCIPLE 2: EAT FOODS
IN AS NATURAL AND FRESH
A STATE AS POSSIBLE

The diet that protected our Paleolithic ancestors from Syndrome X
consisted entirely of natural foods—foods that came directly off
the vine or off the hoof. The more we can replicate that type of
diet—in other words, the more foods we can eat that are close
to how you would find them in the wild—the better protected we
will be.

There are several reasons why a more natural diet is best. As a general rule, the more whole and natural a carbohydrate you eat, the lower your body's glucose and insulin responses will be to that food. In contrast, the more a carbohydrate is processed—that is, the more it is ground into finer and finer forms with less and less of the fiber of the original carbohydrate—the higher your body's glucose and insulin responses will be to that food.

As an example of this rule, consider that:

- An apple causes a lower glucose and insulin response than applesauce.
- Applesauce causes a lower glucose and insulin response than apple juice.
- Apple juice causes a lower glucose and insulin response than apple-juice concentrate.

Each step in processing changes the carbohydrate into a form with a higher glycemic index—one that more rapidly raises glucose and insulin levels higher and higher. The apple—the most natural, intact form of the fruit we can eat—is best in terms of preventing insulin resistance because it is richest in fiber, which slows the entry of glucose into the bloodstream. When you eat natural, unprocessed carbohydrates with all or most of their fiber intact, you take important steps to prevent the development of insulin resistance.

Unprocessed carbohydrates have another big benefit: They are much more nutrient dense than processed carbohydrates. In other words, you get much more of a nutritional bang for your buck with whole-food carbohydrates: They supply greater amounts of nutrients (e.g., vitamins and minerals) relative to their calories or carbohydrates. The more processed carbohydrates are—the further they are removed from their natural state—the lower in nutrients they usually become. For example, brown rice is more nutrient dense than white rice; fresh-cooked beans are more nutrient dense than canned beans; and fresh, just-picked vegetables are more nutrient dense than frozen ones.

The body needs vitamins and minerals to aid the breakdown of carbohydrates and their conversion to energy. Eating nutrient-poor processed carbohydrates, therefore, encourages inefficient carbohydrate metabolism and insulin resistance, while eating nutrient-dense carbohydrates promotes more efficient carbohydrate metabolism and normal insulin function.

There is yet another reason why a diet consisting mostly of natural foods is best: It encourages a dietary potassium-to-sodium ratio

THE POTASSIUM AND SODIUM CONTENT OF SELECTED FOODS

This table shows the potassium and sodium content of natural foods compared with processed foods. Notice how foods in their natural form (in bold type) are low in sodium, contributing less than 140 mg of sodium per serving. They also have potassium-to-sodium ratios above 4:1, which is very desirable. When these same foods are processed, sodium dominates over potassium.

	Potassium	Sodium	Potassium-to-Sodium Ratio
Apple (100 g)	152 mg	1 mg	150.00 [150:1]
Apple pie (100 g)	80 mg	301 mg	0.27 [1:3.7]
Cabbage (100 g)	233 mg	20 mg	12.00 [12:1]
Canned sauerkraut (100 g)	140 mg	747 mg	0.19 [1:5.3]
Cucumber (100 g)	160 mg	6 mg	27.00 [27:1]
Dill pickles (100 g)	200 mg	1,428 mg	0.14 [1:7.2]
Fresh ground beef (100 g)	270 mg	60 mg	4.5 [4.5:1]
McDonald's hamburger (102 g)	142 mg	490 mg	0.27 [1:3.7]
Low-salt tuna in water (184 g)	487 mg	72 mg	6.8 [6.8:1]
Regular tuna in water (184 g)	487 mg	865 mg	0.56 [1:1.7]

Source: Adapted from *The High Blood Pressure Solution,* by Richard D. Moore, M.D., Ph.D., published by Healing Arts Press, an imprint of Inner Traditions International, Rochester, VT 05767. Copyright © 1993 Richard Moore. Reprinted with permission of the publisher.

more in keeping with the ratio our bodies were designed for. Virtually all natural foods have a high potassium-to-sodium ratio—in other words, large amounts of potassium and small amounts of sodium. By contrast, as foods become more and more processed and altered for preservation, they lose potassium and gain sodium, reversing their potassium-to-sodium ratio. A poor potassium-to-sodium ratio in the diet may interfere with normal cell function, and it is associated with an increased risk for Syndrome X–associated conditions, such as high blood pressure, cardiovascular disease, stroke, and cancer.

ANTI-X PRINCIPLE 3: EMPHASIZE NONSTARCHY VEGETABLES IN YOUR DIET

The primary types of carbohydrates eaten in the Paleolithic diet were *nonstarchy* vegetables. Their modern-day equivalents include lettuce, spinach, celery, and broccoli. To prevent and reverse insulin resistance, these and other nonstarchy vegetables should be the primary types of carbohydrates in our diet, too.

EXAMPLES OF NONSTARCHY VEGETABLES

All lettuces and greens	Green, red, and Chinese cabbage
Asparagus	Mushrooms
Bok choy	Spinach
Broccoli	Sweet and hot peppers
Cauliflower	Tomatoes
Celery	Yellow wax beans and green beans
Cucumber	Zucchini and summer squash

Nonstarchy vegetables differ from *starchy* vegetables (which usually are root vegetables such as potatoes and carrots), in that they are substantially lower in carbohydrates (and calories). The "carbohydrate density" of a food—that is, the total amount of digestible carbohydrates—is very important. The more digestible carbohydrates you eat, the more insulin your body will ultimately produce in response. You can eat significantly more nonstarchy vegetables than starchy vegetables because the former contain fewer digestible carbohydrates. Nonstarchy vegetables have two other benefits. They are very nutrient dense—that is, they supply a lot of nutrients (such as vitamins and minerals) with proportionately few calories. Nonstarchy vegetables are also digested slowly and have a low glycemic index—that is, they cause minimal rises in glucose and insulin levels.

ANTI-X PRINCIPLE 4: KEEP YOUR INTAKE OF NATURAL CARBOHYDRATE-DENSE FOODS MODERATE OR LOW

To prevent Syndrome X, natural carbohydrate-dense foods—such as whole grains, starchy vegetables, legumes, and fruits—should be eaten in relatively small amounts. These foods should also be consumed with protein and fat to buffer their glucose-elevating effect. To reverse Syndrome X, more drastic action is needed. At least for a while, these carbohydrate-dense foods should be completely avoided.

This dietary principle is often one of the hardest for many people to understand because they assume that all natural foods must be healthy foods. That is not always the case.

Bear in mind that people, throughout most of their evolution, ate few foods that were rich sources of carbohydrates. Whole grains, legumes, and root vegetables (e.g., potatoes, carrots) probably were rarely eaten, if at all, by Paleolithic people. The fruits that were eaten in Paleolithic times were much less sweet than the fruit of today, and fruits were not eaten in cold climates and during cold seasons because they were not available. Large amounts of carbohydrate-dense foods—natural or processed—are incompatible with our genetic heritage and increase the risk of Syndrome X.

SIMPLIFIED GLYCEMIC INDEX

The *glycemic index* is a scale based on the rate of glucose entry into the bloodstream after a specific carbohydrate is eaten. The lower the glycemic rating of a carbohydrate, the lower (or more desirable) your body's glucose and insulin responses will be to that carbohydrate. Diets high in high-glycemic foods lead to insulin resistance. Diets emphasizing foods that are moderate or low on the glycemic index, in contrast, help protect against insulin resistance.

High-Glycemic Foods
(which cause sharp rises in blood-sugar and insulin levels)

- Most grains and grain products, such as bread (both whole wheat and white)
- Breakfast cereals, such as corn flakes and muesli
- Instant and quick-cooking cereals and grains
- Grain-based snack foods, such as corn chips
- Honey and table sugar

- Most cookies, candies, and candy bars
- Corn and potatoes
- Bananas and most dried fruits

Moderate-Glycemic Foods
(which cause moderate rises in blood-sugar and insulin levels)

- Yams and sweet potatoes
- Regular (slow-cooking) oatmeal
- Many legumes (canned kidney beans, pinto beans, navy beans, peas)

Low-Glycemic Foods
(which induce low blood-sugar and insulin responses)

- Other legumes (fresh-cooked kidney beans, lentils, black-eyed peas, chickpeas, lima beans)
- Dairy products, such as milk and yogurt
- Many fruits, such as peaches, grapes, cherries, plums, and grapefruit
- Nonstarchy vegetables, such as lettuce, broccoli, and celery

As you can see from the glycemic index, starchy vegetables and whole grains rank higher and are less desirable than nonstarchy vegetables because starchy vegetables and whole grains raise glucose and insulin levels higher and more quickly. Numerous studies have found that eating foods low on the glycemic index improves glucose tolerance and insulin function. So, even though starchy vegetables and whole grains may be more nutritious than white bread and more complex in structure than simple sugars, they cause rises in blood sugar and insulin levels very similar to those caused by refined carbohydrates. Therefore, avoid these items when trying to reverse insulin resistance, and eat them only moderately when simply trying to prevent it.

Legumes, such as beans and peas, do not rank high on the glycemic index, but they are carbohydrate dense, like whole grains and starchy vegetables. The total amount of insulin your body produces depends on the carbohydrate density of the foods you consume. The more carbohydrates you eat, the more insulin your body will produce. So, while legumes do not cause a quick, high rise in insulin levels, they do promote sustained insulin production. The more legumes, whole grains, and starchy vegetables you eat, the more insulin you will produce. As we explained in Chapter 4, elevated insulin levels are a problem all by themselves, and the more insulin your body produces, the more weight you'll tend to gain.

In contrast, nonstarchy vegetables have *four to ten times less* carbohydrates than do grain-based foods, starchy vegetables, and legumes. You can, therefore, eat a lot of nonstarchy vegetables without developing insulin-related health problems. On the other hand, you need to limit your intake of starchy vegetables, whole grains, and legumes to avoid developing problems. If you already have signs of insulin resistance, you need to avoid these foods to prevent a worsening of your condition.

CONTROLLING YOUR INTAKE OF CARBOHYDRATE-DENSE FOODS

To prevent Syndrome X, limit yourself to no more than a total of four servings of starches and fruits each day. Emphasize fruits over starches—that is, over whole grains, legumes, and starchy vegetables. For best results, consume no more than two servings per day from starches.

Serving sizes for starches are

> 1 slice whole-grain bread
> ½ cup oatmeal or ½ cup other cooked whole grains
> 1 small or ½ large baked potato
> 1 medium sweet potato or yam
> ½ cup beans, peas, or lentils
> ½ cup corn
> 1 cup carrots

Serving sizes for fruits are

> 1 small apple, orange, or pear
> 1 medium peach or nectarine
> 2 small plums
> 1 cup berries (any type), grapes, or watermelon chunks
> 1 kiwi
> ½ banana
> ¼ melon (cantaloupe, honeydew, etc.)
> ½ cup pineapple

Generally speaking, fruits rank lower on the glycemic index and are lower in carbohydrate density than are starchy vegetables, whole grains, and legumes. There are a few exceptions to these rules, though: Bananas, dried fruits, and most fruit juices rank quite high on the glycemic index. These foods also are carbohydrate dense and, as a consequence, promote more insulin production than do lower-carbohydrate fruits such as strawberries and grapefruit. Other fruits can be enjoyed, as well, but because they are more carbohydrate dense than nonstarchy vegetables, their overconsumption can lead to elevated glucose and insulin levels. Fruits, therefore, probably should be limited to two servings per day.

CARBOHYDRATE DENSITY OF SOME FOODS

The carbohydrate density (CD) of a food refers to the *digestible* carbohydrates, which is calculated from the total carbohydrate (TC) content minus the fiber (–F) content of that food. The amount of insulin your body produces ultimately depends on the CD of the food you eat. To avoid overeating carbohydrates and gaining weight, emphasize low-carbohydrate foods, such as nonstarchy vegetables and fruits, which are toward the bottom of the following list.

Food	Serving Size	CD	TC – F
Plain sheet cake with frosting	⅑ of a cake	71	71 – <1
Apple pie	⅙ of a pie	51	54 – 3
Fast-food bean burrito	1	50	57 – 7
Plain sheet cake	⅑ of a cake	48	48 – <1
Baked potato with skin	4¾" by 2⅓"	47	51 – 4
Pretzels	10 thin twists	45	47 – 2
Peanut butter and jelly	One sandwich on whole-wheat bread	44	51 – 7
Low-fat yogurt with fruit added	1 cup	43	43 – <1
Cola	12 ounces	40	40 – <1

(continued)

Food	Serving Size	CD	TC – F
Spaghetti, enriched	1 cup	38	40 – 2
Cheese pizza	⅛ of 15″ pizza	37	39 – 2
Spaghetti with tomato sauce	1 cup	36	38 – 2
Cooked chickpeas	1 cup	35	45 – 10
Plain bagel	1	35	36 – 1
French bread	2 slices	34	36 – 2
Whole-wheat spaghetti	1 cup	32	37 – 5
Avocado, cheese, tomato, and lettuce	One sandwich on whole-wheat bread	32	39 – 7
Apple juice	1 cup	29	29 – <1
Bread stuffing	1 cup	26	30 – 4
Banana	1 whole medium	25	27 – 2
Cooked black beans	1 cup	24	40 – 16
Grapefruit juice	1 cup	22	22 – <1
Whole-wheat bread	2 slices	22	26 – 4
Apple butter	2 tablespoons	17	17 – <1
Butternut squash	1 cup cubes	15	21 – 6
Tomato sauce	1 cup	14	18 – 4
Milk	1 cup	11	11 – <1
Peach	1 medium	9	10 – 1
Grapes	10	9	9 – <1
Pink grapefruit	1/2	8	9 – 1
Strawberries	1 cup	6	10 – 4
Tomatoes	1 cup	6	8 – 2
Asparagus	1 cup	6	8 – 2
Green beans	1 cup	6	10 – 4
Whole almonds	1 ounce	4	6 – 2
Cooked broccoli	1 cup	4	8 – 4
Bok choy	1 cup	1	3 – 2
Lettuce, romaine	1 cup	1	1 – <1

ANTI-X PRINCIPLE 5: AVOID SOFT DRINKS, FRUIT JUICES, ALCOHOL, AND OTHER HIGHLY PROCESSED DRINKS

Paleolithic people drank little or no alcohol, and they didn't drink glucose-raising soft drinks, sweetened drinks, fruit juices, and caffeine-containing beverages at all. They drank the only beverage that's a nutrient all by itself—water. To prevent and reverse Syndrome X, we need to mimic this behavior as best we can.

Of utmost importance is to avoid soft drinks. These beverages, which were developed only about a century ago, are, for all practical purposes, the equivalent of liquid candy. As concentrated sources of sugars, they quickly raise glucose and insulin to high levels. They are, therefore, one of the greatest contributors to insulin resistance among North Americans, especially in children and teenagers.

Also avoid fruit drinks and fruit juices. Although fruit beverages may seem healthy, they contain the sugars from pounds of fruit without any of the glucose-regulating fiber. Fruit drinks, which contain some fruit juice and lots of sugar, are even worse. Both types of drinks assault glucose and insulin control.

The research on alcohol is a mixed bag: Wine has been found beneficial for heart health, but alcohol in general is metabolized by the body as a carbohydrate and can contribute to glucose- and insulin-related health problems. To understand what alcohol does in the body, just think of someone with a "beer belly." A beer belly is a clear sign of insulin resistance caused by too many carbohydrates that raise glucose and insulin levels quickly. Alcohol, in other words, acts very much like sugar in the body. It also damages brain and liver cells and can lead to a fatty liver that doesn't process fats properly. So, it's probably best to avoid alcohol, particularly if you show signs of severe insulin resistance.

The most healthful drink, of course, is the one our bodies thirst for—water, preferably filtered or bottled. In moderation, sparkling water, herbal teas, black tea, and green tea are other acceptable choices.

ANTI-X DIET PRINCIPLE 6: AVOID COMMON VEGETABLE OILS, AND USE OLIVE OIL INSTEAD

Just as you should avoid refined carbohydrates to prevent the development or progression of insulin resistance, you should also avoid most vegetable oils, which have been manufactured on a

massive scale only during the past century. Corn, soybean, safflower, sunflower, and cottonseed oil are all high in omega-6 fatty
acids, which have been promoted since the 1970s as a "healthy"
alternative to saturated fats (found in meat and lard). However,
omega-6 fatty acids are not healthy in the quantities Americans eat
them.

Omega-6 fatty acids and omega-3 fatty acids are essential fats
needed for health. People do best consuming them in the balance
humans evolved on—between 1:1 and 4:1. The current ratio of
omega-6 to omega-3 fatty acids in the U.S. diet ranges from 20:1 to
30:1. This ratio is seriously unbalanced and contributes significantly
to insulin resistance and obesity. Research has found that feeding
animals a diet high in omega-6 oils results in insulin resistance.

A high ratio of omega-6-to-omega-3 fatty acids may promote
obesity, as well. When mice prone to diabetes and obesity are
raised on a diet high in omega-6-rich soybean oil (an oil that's
found in a wide range of processed convenience foods), they end
up the fattest—even fatter than those fed a high-lard (saturated
fat) diet. However, when these mice are fed a diet containing high
amounts of omega-3-rich fish oils, they become the leanest. This
same phenomenon is just starting to be seen in research with
humans. One study found that people whose muscle cells contain
low levels of omega-3 fatty acids and high levels of omega-6 fatty
acids are more likely to be insulin resistant and obese.

By asking you to avoid oils rich in omega-6 fatty acids, we are
not asking you to eat a fat-free diet. To the contrary, a fat-free diet is
inevitably a high-carbohydrate diet that promotes insulin resistance. In addition to reducing your intake of omega-6 fatty acids,
there are two more crucial ways to manage your fatty acids. One is
to use unrefined or cold-pressed extra-virgin olive oil as your primary oil in salads and cooking. Olive oil is low in omega-6 fatty
acids and rich in omega-9 monounsaturated fatty acids, which do
not compete with omega-3 fatty acids in the body. The second way
to manage fatty acids, which we describe in the next principle, is to
increase your intake of omega-3 fatty acids.

Diets high in omega-9 monounsaturated fatty acids have been
found very helpful for diabetics. Monounsaturated fats increase
levels of the good HDL cholesterol and inhibit the oxidation of
the bad LDL cholesterol. Substituting monounsaturated fats for
carbohydrates also improves insulin sensitivity. Thus, monounsaturated fats can be helpful for those with mild insulin resistance, as
well.

Olive oil is particularly healthful because it has mild antithrombotic (anticlotting) properties. It isn't surprising, therefore, that Mediterranean people, who have a diet high in olive oil, have a lower incidence of heart disease and stroke, compared with people in other regions—and Mediterranean people live longer, too. For all of these reasons, to both prevent and reverse insulin resistance, make an important oil change—olive oil instead of omega-6-rich vegetable oils. It is okay, by the way, to buy convenience foods that contain monounsaturated-rich canola oil, too, but make a point of using olive oil as your primary cooking oil.

ANTI-X PRINCIPLE 7: ENRICH YOUR DIET WITH OMEGA-3 FATS WHENEVER YOU CAN

The body needs the omega-3 fatty acids to produce flexible cell membranes. Such membranes contain large numbers of insulin receptors and are more receptive and responsive to insulin. Without sufficient omega-3 fatty acids (especially one particular type, called DHA [docosahexaenoic acid], found in fish oils), the membranes are not as flexible, and insulin resistance can develop.

Eating a diet rich in omega-3 fatty acids not only can help prevent insulin resistance and Syndrome X, but also can help reverse these conditions. In one study, 55 people diagnosed with Syndrome X ate a diet high in omega-3-rich fish. A year later, lab tests showed they had become less insulin resistant—and they also had lower body weight, triglycerides, and blood pressure.

In another study, diabetics were asked to eat a diet relatively high in omega-3 fatty acids and monounsaturated oils. After one year, people eating this diet were more sensitive to insulin and less insulin resistant; they had reductions in blood pressure, fasting glucose, and triglycerides; and they had increases in HDL cholesterol. This study showed that eating a diet that emphasizes omega-3 and monounsaturated fats is very effective medicine against Syndrome X.

Increasing your intake of omega-3 fatty acids is important for another reason: It protects against one of the main consequences of Syndrome X—namely, cardiovascular disease. Supplementing the diet with small amounts of omega-3 fatty acids reduces *platelet aggregation* (the tendency of blood clots to form), even in diabetics. This in turn reduces the risk of heart attack and stroke.

Unfortunately, sources of omega-3 fatty acids in the typical U.S. diet are scarce to nonexistent. The easiest way to improve your omega-3 fatty acid intake is to eat cold-water fish, such as salmon, trout, and tuna two to three times a week. If you don't like fish or can't eat it that often, don't despair. There are numerous delicious ways to increase the omega-3 fatty acid content of your diet, as you'll read in the following suggestions.

WAYS TO INCREASE OMEGA-3 FATTY ACIDS IN YOUR DIET

- Eat cold-water fish, such as salmon, trout, tuna, sardines, herring, and anchovies. Eating these fish just once a week helps reduce your risk of a heart attack.
- Add omega-3-rich flaxseed oil to salad dressings, and drizzle it on top of cooked cereals and vegetables.
- Add chopped walnuts or ground flaxseed on top of cereals or salads, or in baked goods, or eat a few walnuts as snacks.
- Try to find omega-3-enriched eggs and meats. A number of egg producers are now using a mash that has been enriched with omega-3 fatty acids, either from fish meal or flaxseeds; some also contain added vitamin E.
- When you're lucky enough to find it, choose meat and milk products from free-range animals that eat omega-3-rich grass and insects (rather than those fattened up on omega-6-rich grains).
- When available, try game meat such as venison, buffalo, or game birds; they have a fatty-acid profile more closely resembling the fatty-acid profiles of the wild meats our ancestors ate.
- Look for other omega-3-enriched foods. One such product is Millina's Healthy Kitchen organic pasta sauces, with added omega-3 nutrients (and no fishy taste).
- Eat your veggies—specifically, the dark-green, leafy ones. Good sources of omega-3 fatty acids include romaine lettuce, mesclun mixed greens, arugula, kale, collards, mustard greens, and Swiss chard.
- If you don't like fatty fish or any of the other food ideas listed here, consider taking omega-3-containing fish-oil supplements (with vitamin E to prevent rancidity).

ANTI-X PRINCIPLE 8: STEER CLEAR OF TRANS-FATTY ACIDS

In addition to avoiding omega-6-rich vegetable oils, it is also of paramount importance to avoid trans-fatty acids. Trans-fatty acids were first produced commercially at the start of the twentieth century, during the hydrogenation of oils. Today, trans-fatty acids are widespread in the typical North American diet: They are found in margarine, deep-fried foods, and foods that contain partially hydrogenated oils—a wide array of convenience foods, including salad dressings, crackers, breads, cookies, and pastries.

Trans-fatty acids promote insulin resistance and a variety of health problems in the body because they are shaped differently than the polyunsaturated fatty acids from which they are made. Essentially, they act like misfits. They crowd out essential fats from the cell membranes and interfere with the conversion of shorter-chain fatty acids into longer ones.

One consequence is that fewer long-chain fatty acids are incorporated into cell membranes, making the membranes less fluid and reducing the number and sensitivity of insulin receptors. Trans-fatty acids, therefore, promote not only insulin resistance, but also the health problems that accompany insulin resistance. In one study, women who ate margarine four or more times per week had a higher than normal risk of three of the symptoms of Syndrome X: high triglycerides, low HDL cholesterol, and high total cholesterol.

Trans-fatty acids also appear to promote obesity. Animal experiments have found that trans-fatty acids increase the size of fat cells, and large fat cells have fewer insulin receptors and store more fat than normal fat cells.

What's even worse is that diets with a lot of trans-fatty acids double the risk of heart disease. It has been estimated that each year, 30,000 premature heart-disease deaths in the United States can be attributed to the intake of trans-fatty acids. If you want to prevent insulin resistance and the very serious complications associated with it, you should substantially reduce your intake of trans-fatty acids by avoiding fried foods (e.g., fried chicken, french fries) and foods that contain partially hydrogenated oils (e.g., margarine, vegetable shortening, many microwavable and TV dinners, crackers, and other convenience foods).

ANTI-X PRINCIPLE 9: EAT PROTEIN AT EVERY MEAL AND SNACK

Our Paleolithic ancestors averaged slightly more than 30 percent protein in their diet; the average U.S. resident eats a diet with only 12 percent protein.

Protein plays many critical roles in the body, not the least of which is to stimulate the production of glucagon. *Glucagon* is a hormone that opposes insulin and that allows the body to burn stored fat and stored carbohydrates (called glycogen) for energy. Glucagon, in other words, helps counter excessive insulin production, stimulate fat burning in the body, and maintain the tight balance of blood glucose required for the brain and body to function properly. If you want to prevent or reverse insulin resistance, feel good, and lose or maintain weight, it is absolutely essential that you consume adequate amounts of protein throughout the day.

PROTEIN SOURCES

Animal foods—chicken, turkey, fish, seafood, red meat, game meats, eggs, and low-fat cheese—are all rich sources of protein. A good serving size per meal for most people is 3 to 4 ounces—about the size of a deck of cards.

The very best types of animal protein are wild game meats such as venison, rabbit, and game birds. These meats are high in protein, low in overall fat and saturated fat, and rich in micronutrients. They most resemble the type of protein Paleolithic people ate. Also extremely beneficial and healthy are meats from free-ranging animals that eat green grass and insects; organic meats from animals that are not treated with hormones, steroids, or antibiotics; eggs from free-range chickens; and eggs from chickens fed omega-3-rich flaxseed or fish meal.

The best types of commercial meat are fresh, unprocessed chicken and turkey, and unprocessed lean cuts of lamb and beef. Deep-fried meats and processed meat products—such as sausage, bacon, hot dogs, and luncheon meats—are very different from the types of protein Paleolithic people ate; they are the most unhealthy and should be avoided.

Legumes contain some protein but they're far higher in carbohydrates than in protein.

Nuts and seeds also contain some protein, but they are significantly higher in fat than protein. The fat they contain is beneficial—

mostly monounsaturated fat—so small amounts of nuts and seeds make healthful snacks. Seeds are slightly more desirable than nuts because they generally tend to be higher in protein.

Cheese was not eaten at all by Paleolithic people, and most cheeses are higher in fat than in protein. However, low-fat cheeses, such as part-skim mozzarella, feta, and low-fat or fat-free cottage cheese, have greater or equal amounts of protein compared to fat. In other words, they have a protein-to-fat ratio more supportive of health and the prevention of insulin resistance. Small amounts of low-fat cheeses, therefore, can be included as good, convenient sources of protein, for variety in the diet.

Unfortunately, many people do not think much about food until they are very hungry, and then they grab something quick to eat (which is almost always something that contains ready-to-eat processed carbohydrates). They go through the day eating this way, although they might sit down to a decent meal with some protein at dinner. It's simply impossible, though, to eat the daily amount of protein you need for health in one sitting. Furthermore, when you eat protein only at one meal—such as at dinnertime—it means you're eating too many carbohydrates at other meals to keep glucose and insulin levels in healthy ranges. Eating this way is a prescription for Syndrome X.

To change your habits so they are Anti-X in nature, you have to think of protein as more than a dietary afterthought: Protein needs to be a centerpiece of your diet. Your focus should be on eating small amounts of high-quality protein throughout the day, preferably at every meal and snack. Then you should balance the protein with a small to moderate amount of carbohydrates (depending on your condition). Doing this leads to healthy blood-sugar balance, which in turn helps both prevent and reverse insulin resistance, weight problems, and Syndrome X.

Putting This Chapter into Practice

Whether you are trying to prevent or reverse Syndrome X, it is important to eat as many fresh, unprocessed foods as possible, with the emphasis on fowl, fish, and vegetables. It is also crucial to avoid refined foods, such as breads, pastas, pastries, candies, and cooking oils (with the exception of olive oil).

- To prevent Syndrome X, eat no more than small to moderate amounts of natural carbohydrate-dense foods—such as whole grains, starchy vegetables, legumes, and fruits. Make a point of eating these carbohydrates with protein and fat to buffer their glucose-boosting effect.

- To reverse Syndrome X, completely avoid carbohydrate-dense foods—even if they are natural—until insulin-related health problems diminish. Your only sources of carbohydrates should be non-starchy vegetables.

CHAPTER 8

Navigating through Restaurants and Supermarkets

Now that you understand the principles of the Anti-X diet, the next step is to put them into practice in your life. The first two places to begin are in restaurants and in supermarkets—where virtually all of us make our initial food choices.

The foods that most of us have selected in the past few decades have been the exact ones that set the stage for Syndrome X. As just one example, the intake of grain-based foods has skyrocketed since the late 1970s. Whether chosen in fast-food restaurants, four-star restaurants, or at home, foods such as pasta, bread, pizza, rice, sandwiches, and pretzels are made primarily or entirely of refined carbohydrates, the same type that greatly increases the risk of insulin resistance. It isn't surprising, therefore, that the more people have selected foods such as pasta and bread in restaurants and supermarkets, the more common obesity and other glucose-related disorders have become.

If you make bad food choices in restaurants and supermarkets, you simply cannot follow the Anti-X diet. If you take the time to learn to be a savvy food consumer, though, you will lay the groundwork for a diet that not only reverses insulin resistance but also prevents it throughout your lifetime.

DEVELOPING RESTAURANT SAVVY

In the fast-paced world we live in, we often don't have the time to cook three meals from scratch at home each day, so we let others do the cooking for us, often by eating in restaurants. This makes

life simpler and more convenient, but it also can set us up for
insulin-related weight problems and health problems if we're not
careful about the foods we get.

We cover the subject of ordering foods in restaurants first because more Americans than ever eat out. In fact, many busy people
eat out more than they eat in. Knowing how to get healthy, balanced meals when eating out, therefore, is a survival skill virtually
all of us need to learn if we want to prevent or reverse Syndrome X.

The Basic Rule to Follow When Ordering in Restaurants

The basic rule to follow when ordering in virtually any restaurant is
this:

> Select a serving of any type of animal protein—that is, fish, seafood,
> chicken, turkey, lean red meats, or game meat—that is baked, broiled,
> steamed, stewed, sautéed, or poached. Then select at least two servings
> of vegetables to accompany the protein.

A word of caution: Some vegetables raise blood glucose levels
so quickly that they should be counted as two vegetables in the
basic Anti-X diet. These vegetables include a baked potato, a cup
of carrots, and half a cup of corn, beets, peas, or beans. Otherwise,
the sky's the limit in terms of mixing and matching vegetables.
Some examples of combinations to order are broccoli and green
beans, a double order of broccoli, a double order of a vegetable
medley, a large salad with assorted vegetables, and asparagus, mushrooms, and a side salad.

Ideally, the protein you eat should make up about one third of
your plate, and the vegetables should take up at least two thirds of
your plate. In some restaurants, this is difficult to achieve, but the
closer you can come to this basic formula, the more Anti-X your
meal will be.

It is easiest to follow the preceding guideline if you visit restaurants that cook food to order (in contrast to fast-food restaurants,
which generally serve food *their* way). It is also important to ask the
waiter questions about how food is prepared and to learn to pick
and choose from the menu. You will find that most restaurants—
other than the fast-food variety—are really very accommodating to
what their customers want. Keep in mind that if a particular item is
listed somewhere on the menu, you should be able to get it, even
though it may not be listed with the particular entree you want. For
example, if you see a chicken entree you want that's listed with

pasta, and elsewhere on the menu, you see green beans listed with another entree and a side spinach salad listed with another one, you should be able to combine the items you want from the three different listings and get the chicken with green beans and a spinach salad instead of with pasta. By honing this creative combining skill and developing it to a fine art, you can make your own individualized Anti-X meals while letting others do the cooking for you.

Another point to keep in mind: Many restaurants serve way too much food per meal. Serving portions of meat often are excessively large. Don't be afraid to ask for a "doggie bag" or box to take food home with you. Extra food from restaurant meals makes great leftovers for lunch, dinner, or a snack the next day.

Suggestions for Ordering in Different Kinds of Restaurants

Part of the fun of eating out is getting to experience something new or different from the usual routine at home. Whether the restaurant offers a different ambience, a different kind of food, or entertainment and sociability, it's often just plain fun to eat out.

Sometimes, when we're busy, eating out isn't fun; it's just convenient. Grabbing something quick is often the only way to keep ourselves going amidst the deadlines, time pressures, and obligations most of us have.

In either case—whether you grab a quick meal at a fast-food restaurant or enjoy a leisurely meal at an upscale ethnic eatery—you cannot just order foods blindly. There are hidden obstacles to Anti-X eating in every type of restaurant, and you need to understand these obstacles and learn how to navigate around them so that the fun and convenience of eating out doesn't sabotage your health. The tips that follow do just that; they teach you how to employ the basic Anti-X diet principles in all the different restaurants you visit. First, we offer some suggestions for breakfast, lunch, and dinner in basic North American–style and hotel restaurants, then we cover good lunch and dinner choices in a variety of ethnic restaurants.

North American–Style and Hotel Restaurants

FOR BREAKFAST. You need to be especially careful when ordering breakfast because refined carbohydrates and sugar-laced foods abound on the typical breakfast menu. These include pastries, croissants, and muffins; bagels, toast, English muffins, and jam; pancakes, waffles, and syrup; fruit-flavored yogurt; and granola and other sweetened cereals.

To navigate around these obstacles, think protein. Protein-rich eggs are almost always the best choice on the menu; you can have them prepared virtually any way. To get some beneficial vegetables into your diet, peruse the menu and look for omelets that contain vegetables or for scrambled-egg-vegetable combinations—for example, a spinach, onion, and mushroom omelet, or huevos rancheros (Mexican-style eggs with tomatoes, peppers, onions, chiles, and often a little cheese). If you don't see anything like this, don't be afraid to ask your server whether the kitchen staff can make a combination such as this; it's usually easy enough for the chef to do. If you want some cheese with the eggs, try to choose low-fat cheeses such as mozzarella, provolone, or Swiss, or just tell the server to "go easy on the cheese" to avoid getting more fat than protein. By the way, after decades of antiegg hysteria, eggs have been redeemed: Moderate consumption of eggs has been found not to raise cholesterol levels, and eggs are one of the best sources of low-fat protein around.

Other protein foods that work well in a pinch are low-fat cottage cheese, Canadian bacon, turkey sausage, and lox or smoked salmon; however, several of these also contain nitrite additives that can convert to tumor-promoting nitrosamines in the body. To protect yourself from this hazard, we recommend eating vitamin-C-rich fruits when you eat these foods. If you can't do so, take vitamin C and vitamin E supplements. Vitamins C and E help prevent the formation of nitrosamines.

Unfortunately, very few other sources of protein typically are offered for breakfast. You may want to try asking for a special request of something like a broiled chicken breast for breakfast. Although such breakfast orders may seem a little strange at first, they are a great way to start the day—and restaurants in many hotels typically accommodate simple special requests such as these.

Fresh fruit is a very healthful complement to protein at breakfast. The best fruits to order—those lowest in carbohydrates and lowest on the glycemic index—are half a grapefruit, some cantaloupe or melon, or a bowl of strawberries. Avoid fruit juices, such as orange juice. Even though juices are popular drinks in the morning, they provide all the sugars from pounds and pounds of fresh fruit without any of the glucose-regulating fiber; this is a recipe for insulin-related health problems.

If you are following a prevention or maintenance-type Anti-X diet moderate in carbohydrates, slow-cooked oatmeal can be a good choice for breakfast. Be sure to avoid brown sugar or maple syrup toppings for the oatmeal, though, and ask for fresh fruit or raisins instead. Balance out the meal with some eggs or a piece of lean ham or Canadian bacon.

> ### EXAMPLE OF AN ANTI-X BREAKFAST
> Spinach, onion, and mushroom omelet
> ½ grapefruit

FOR LUNCH AND DINNER. If the menu at the restaurant offers mostly burgers and sandwiches, simply order the meat or chicken without a bun and with veggies and a veggie salad or a fruit salad as a replacement.

There also are usually a variety of good salad and meat combinations to choose from, ranging from chef salad to chicken Caesar salad. The bad news about ordering a salad is that many of the commercially prepared salad dressings offered in restaurants are similar to those found in the average grocery store—in other words, they often contain hidden sources of sugar, additives, hydrogenated oils, and processed omega-6-rich oils such as soybean oil. There are several ways around these obstacles. One, you can ask for olive oil and vinegar, or olive oil and lemon wedges; these are the healthiest salad dressings to order. Another option is to order any *regular* salad dressing "on the side," use it sparingly, and perhaps thin out the dressing you use with lemon juice or lemon juice and olive oil. It's important not to order a fat-free dressing; the fat that's missing from these dressings is typically replaced with extra sugars.

Processed carbohydrates—which you should avoid—are routinely served in restaurants unless you specifically ask that they not be. Here are a few tips:

- Always order salads without the croutons.
- At salad bars, avoid carbohydrate-rich salads such as pasta salad, macaroni salad, and potato salad.
- If something you order comes with one of these carbohydrate-dense salads, ask for a vegetable or fruit salad instead.
- When you order lunch or dinner, ask your server not to bring bread to your table; this way you won't be tempted to grab glucose-raising refined carbohydrates. If you find yourself hungry while waiting for meals or while watching others at your table eat bread, carry a bag of any type of nuts in your

purse or briefcase with you, and snack on these while you're waiting for your entree to arrive.

In terms of entrees, it is usually easy in a hotel or North American–style restaurant to get some type of poultry or meat entree with vegetables and a nice, fresh salad. Various sauces—from salsa to pesto sauce to garlic butter—can be included with these entrees. However, avoid entrees that come with glazes, barbecue sauces, fruit sauces, honey-based sauces, or a restaurant's own "special," "secret," or "sweet" sauce. The main ingredient in these types of sauces is often sugar.

A great entree to order is fresh fish. Many people don't like to cook, or don't know how to cook, fish at home, so treating yourself to fish when you eat out is a good way to get something different and delicious that also offers extra protection against insulin resistance and its complications. (Remember: Eating omega-3-rich fatty fish just once a week helps lower the risk of heart attack.)

FOR DESSERT. In terms of dessert, you need to get into the habit of "just saying no" to it. If you have cravings for carbohydrates, avoiding dessert may seem difficult at first, but it gets easier and easier the more you follow the Anti-X diet.

If you are like most people on the Anti-X diet, your cravings will subside and you'll probably find yourself not wanting or needing desserts. In the early stages of the diet particularly, it is important to remind yourself that virtually all desserts are full of refined sugars and other refined carbohydrates, and they are often high in fat—a very dangerous combination for insulin-related health problems. To really overcome Syndrome X, you need to get out of the habit of thinking you need desserts to finish off meals; the meals you order should be delicious and satisfying enough by themselves.

Another option for dessert is to order a bowl of berries or a fruit salad. Even if you don't see fruit on the menu, don't hesitate to ask for it. Most good restaurants have fruit in the kitchen to use for garnishes or in other desserts; they usually are more than willing to serve it as a substitute dessert.

With all that being said, you don't have to be perfect all the time if you regularly eat according to the principles of the Anti-X diet. A bite of a rich-tasting but not overly sweet dessert on an occasional basis isn't so bad (unless you have severe insulin resistance or diabetes) as long as you eat plenty of protein with your meal and as long as your overall diet is moderate to low in carbohydrates. Human nature is such that we always seem to yearn for the things we can't have, so don't restrict yourself to such an extent that you end up bingeing on sugar. On the exceptional basis—say, a holiday or birthday—choose desserts wisely, share them with several friends, and keep your carbohydrate intake for the day as low as possible. If you end up eating more carbohydrates than you should have one day, the important thing is not to berate yourself, but to get back on the Anti-X diet as soon possible.

> ### EXAMPLE OF A NORTH AMERICAN–STYLE ANTI-X MEAL
> Roast chicken with herbs (skin removed)
> Green beans
> Steamed broccoli with butter
> Bowl of strawberries with a dab of cream

Seafood Restaurants

These are great places to visit for variety in your diet. You can try many different types of healthful fish and shellfish that you may not regularly eat at home. Fish that make especially good choices—those that are particularly rich in beneficial omega-3 fatty acids—are:

Anchovies	King salmon
Atlantic cod	Mackerel
Atlantic salmon	Rainbow trout
Haddock	Tuna
Halibut	

In most seafood restaurants, fish comes with potatoes or rice, vegetables, and a salad. Potatoes and rice raise glucose and insulin levels very quickly, so you should avoid these foods, especially in the early weeks of the Anti-X diet. The way to avoid even being tempted by these foods on your plate is to ask for a double order of vegetables or a double order of salad as a substitute for these starches.

> ### EXAMPLE OF AN ANTI-X SEAFOOD MEAL
> Green leafy salad topped with baby shrimp
> (dressing on the side, used sparingly)
> Broiled salmon served with cucumber-dill-yogurt sauce
> Double order of vegetable medley

Italian Restaurants

Many people equate Italian food with pasta, but there's a lot more than spaghetti to Italian cooking. When you go Italian, lots of Anti-X choices await you—if you order correctly.

The best selections in Italian restaurants include veal, chicken, fish, or shellfish prepared with plenty of heart-healthy garlic and fresh herbs. Avoid entrees with lots of cheese and heavy tomato sauces, and opt instead for those in thin marinara sauces or in light lemon- or wine-based sauces. Instead of pasta or bread with your meal, ask for a leafy green salad and a steamed artichoke served with a vinaigrette dressing, sautéed spinach, or a medley of flavorful grilled or sautéed vegetables.

EXAMPLE OF AN ANTI-X ITALIAN MEAL

Caesar salad, minus the croutons
(Caesar dressing on the side, used sparingly, and
   olive oil and lemon juice)
Chicken piccata (in a lemon/olive oil/wine sauce)
Eggplant, zucchini, and peppers sautéed with
   garlic and herbs

Greek and Middle Eastern Restaurants

Eating the Anti-X way in Greek and Middle Eastern restaurants means avoiding dishes with honey-based sauces, Greek pastries, rice, pasta, loaf bread, and pita bread. Healthful dishes to try include Mediterranean-style fish (broiled with olive oil, lemon, garlic, and herbs), broiled lamb chops, roast leg of lamb, and souvlaki (skewered lamb, beef, chicken, or shrimp kabobs, with vegetables).

The salads in Mediterranean restaurants are delicious. Choose from traditional Greek salad (with lettuce greens, tomatoes, red onions, olives, feta cheese, herbs, and olive oil and red wine vinegar dressing) or house salads topped with tzatziki sauce (yogurt-cucumber sauce) or garlic-herbed olive oil.

EXAMPLE OF AN ANTI-X GREEK MEAL

Traditional Greek salad
Lamb souvlaki, skewered with green peppers,
   tomatoes, onions, and mushrooms
Green beans stewed in a light tomato-garlic sauce

French or Other Continental Restaurants

In French or other continental restaurants, it is most important to avoid bread, flour-based dishes, potato dishes, and sweet-glazed foods such as duck à l'orange. Look instead for baked, broiled, poached, or steamed meats, poultry, and fish, and ask for the sauces on the side.

Some especially good French and continental selections include poached salmon, sole almondine, *fish en papillote* (fish cooked in its own juices with herbs), *poulet aux fines herbes* (roast chicken with herbs), bouillabaisse, steamed mussels, and a variety of salads including salade niçoise.

> ### EXAMPLE OF AN ANTI-X FRENCH OR OTHER CONTINENTAL MEAL
> Appetizers of steamed mussels with garlic butter
>   and steamed artichoke with vinaigrette dressing
> Sole almondine
> Asparagus with butter

Mexican Restaurants

On a moderate-carbohydrate Anti-X prevention diet, you can order chicken or beef tacos in soft corn tortillas, or a taco salad with chicken or beef and beans in Mexican restaurants. On a lower-carbohydrate diet needed for extra healing, though, you need to navigate around carbohydrate-rich foods such as tortillas, beans, and rice, and go for the lowest-carbohydrate dishes available.

Good selections include red snapper or sea bass prepared Veracruz-style (with tomatoes, peppers, and onions), *camarones al mojo de ajo* (shrimp sautéed in olive oil with garlic), and chicken or beef fajitas (minus the tortillas). It's best to avoid foods with a lot of high-fat cheese and sour cream; try asking for salsa or monounsaturated-rich guacamole on the side for extra flavor. Although not a truly Mexican food, gazpacho, a refreshing cold vegetable soup, is a healthy choice available in many Mexican restaurants.

> ### EXAMPLE OF AN ANTI-X MEXICAN MEAL
> Gazpacho
> Sea bass Veracruz (with tomatoes, peppers, and
>   onions) with salsa and guacamole on the side

Chinese Restaurants

In Chinese restaurants, there are a wide variety of tasty stir-fry dishes to choose from—those that combine chicken, beef, or seafood and abundant vegetables such as broccoli, scallions, garlic, ginger, snow peas, green peppers, bean sprouts, bamboo shoots, water chestnuts, bok choy, and Napa cabbage (Chinese cabbage), and sometimes nuts. Be sure, though, to avoid deep-fried and breaded entrees and sugar-containing hoisin, plum, and sweet-and-sour sauces. Request that no sugar be added to your meal during cooking.

If your meal seems a little bland without any extra sugar, ask for some accompaniments from the kitchen—such as hot mustard, minced garlic, scallions, ginger, or some Chinese five-spice powder—to season your meal with a sugar-free, low-sodium kick. Just as you need to ask that bread not be brought to your table in most other types of restaurants, you need to ask that rice not be brought to your table in Chinese restaurants.

EXAMPLE OF AN ANTI-X CHINESE MEAL

Moo goo gai pan without rice (chicken sautéed with pea pods, bamboo shoots, mushrooms, and carrots)

or

Almond chicken without rice

Japanese Restaurants

Like Chinese restaurants, Japanese restaurants offer a variety of protein and veggie combinations. Good choices are chicken or shrimp prepared hibachi-style with lots of vegetables. Sukiyaki and teriyaki dishes typically contain sugar and are best avoided.

EXAMPLE OF AN ANTI-X JAPANESE MEAL

Hibachi shrimp (with bamboo shoots, onions, Napa cabbage, and bean sprouts) without rice

Sushi and sashimi—if you avoid the rice—are other Japanese selections that can fit into the Anti-X diet. The fish in these dishes is an excellent source of protein and beneficial omega-3 fatty acids, which are in short supply in the typical North American diet. There's one big drawback and danger to these dishes, though: Most of the fish is served raw, so there's a risk of parasitic contamination that can cause severe illness. To eliminate this risk, opt for sushi made from *cooked* shrimp, crab, eel, octopus, or egg. If you enjoy sushi or sashimi made from raw fish and want to eat it knowing there is some risk, we strongly urge you to take precautions. Visit an upscale, higher-priced sushi restaurant where the food is carefully prepared in clean conditions and where the chef is especially skilled in sushi preparation. Also be sure to use some of the wasabi sauce served with these entrees: The horseradish in wasabi has antibacterial and antiparasitic properties.

Fast-Food Restaurants

Most fast-food restaurants, which serve burgers, chicken, fries, and so forth, are best avoided because the foods they serve are major sources of hidden sugar, salt, and nonessential fat. The best fast-food outlets are those that offer "home-style" meals such as rotisserie-cooked chicken and turkey. (Be sure to remove the skin from chicken, though, before eating.) Good choices to go with chicken and turkey entrees include steamed vegetable medley, green beans, and other vegetable dishes, fruit salad, and side salads. Skip the macaroni and cheese and potato side dishes.

> ### EXAMPLE OF AN ANTI-X FAST-FOOD MEAL
> Rotisserie-cooked turkey (without gravy)
> Steamed vegetable medley
> Green beans or side salad

Prepackaged salads and salad bars are offered at some fast-food hamburger chains. These are fairly good choices when you're eating on the run, but avoid the prepackaged salad dressings that come with these salads; they are full of hidden sugars, salt, and unhealthy fats. If you know your schedule requires you to pick up a salad to go, carry along your own healthy sugar-free salad dressing in a two-ounce watertight Tupperware container that you can put in your purse or briefcase.

DEVELOPING SUPERMARKET SAVVY

Becoming an Anti-X consumer in the supermarket is similar to being an Anti-X diner at restaurants. You need to recognize common obstacles to Anti-X eating, navigate around them, and choose foods that promote glucose and insulin balance.

Choosing healthful foods actually is probably a little easier in supermarkets than in restaurants, though. In restaurants, you give up some control for convenience. That means refined carbohydrates can sometimes unexpectedly end up on your plate because not all the side dishes or key ingredients are always listed on the menu. In supermarkets, refined carbohydrates are found in very specific areas of the stores—specific areas that you can avoid. In addition, you can see (and read the labels of) exactly what you're getting, and you have control over what you buy. Once you become knowledgeable about the basic layout of a supermarket and how to choose the best convenience foods available, you will find Anti-X shopping simpler than your previous way of shopping.

The Basic Rule to Follow When Grocery Shopping

Supermarket design is relatively consistent, and the basic rule to follow when grocery shopping is this: *Shop mostly on the perimeter.* The freshest, healthiest, and most natural foods are on the edges of supermarkets—in the produce, meat and seafood, frozen foods, and egg, dairy, and perishable foods departments. In contrast, convenience foods that have a long shelf life predominate in the center aisles of the supermarket. The vast majority of these foods are made of refined carbohydrates (primarily white flour and white sugar). Many other processed foods in center aisles contain high levels of sodium and additives.

The following diagram shows you the layout of the typical supermarket. Although the products found in each aisle vary slightly from store to store, the general rule of processed convenience foods being in the center of the store holds true in all supermarkets. As you now understand, the more foods are processed, the worse they are for glucose and insulin levels. Processed carbohydrate foods may have a long *shelf life* (a long life on supermarket shelves without going bad), but the more we eat of them, the more they shorten *our* lives. The bottom line is the more quick, jiffy, pre-made foods you buy in the inner aisles of your grocery store, the more you'll be on the fast track to Syndrome X and all the complications that go with it. The more foods you buy along the perimeter of your grocery store, though, the better protected you will be against Syndrome X.

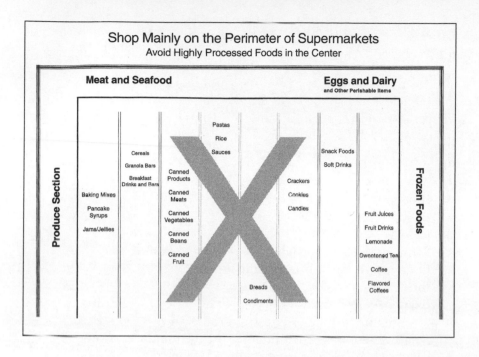

Spending most of your shopping time along the perimeter of your supermarket may take a little getting used to at first, but adopting this practice actually makes shopping easier and also usually quicker and cheaper. To buy foods that come closest to the quality of the foods our distant ancestors thrived on, we recommend shopping in natural-food supermarkets whenever you can. Even in commercial grocery stores, though, an emphasis on shopping along the perimeter will take you a long way toward preventing and reversing insulin resistance. Equally important, though, is to learn how to select the highest-quality natural foods and the most helpful, healthful convenience foods in the supermarket.

What follows is a quick course on the foods to look for and emphasize on a trip to the supermarket. Buying these foods will allow you to follow the Anti-X diet we outline in the next chapter.

Shopping in the Produce Section

One of the basic tenets of Anti-X eating is to emphasize a wide variety of fresh vegetables and, to a lesser extent, fruits in the diet. This means that you should spend much—if not most—of your time grocery shopping in the produce department.

On the basic Anti-X diet, which is moderate in carbohydrates, you can select virtually any fruit or vegetable—even high-glycemic bananas, corn, and potatoes—as long as you select small sizes of these foods and control the portions you eat. Nonstarchy vegetables such as salad greens, broccoli, and green beans, however, should still form the bulk of the produce you buy.

On a lower-carbohydrate Anti-X diet (useful when signs of insulin resistance are pronounced), nonstarchy vegetables and fresh herbs should be the only produce you buy. As a quick reminder, nonstarchy vegetables include:

Asparagus
Bok choy
Broccoli and cauliflower
Celery
Fresh herbs, such as cilantro, parsley, dill, and basil
Green, red, and Chinese cabbage
Mushrooms
Salad greens and other greens of all types (everything from
    romaine lettuce to endive to radicchio)
Salad vegetables (cucumber, radishes, tomatoes, sweet and
    hot peppers, and green onions)
Spinach
Zucchini and summer squash

Especially Healthful Vegetables to Buy

Some vegetables have medicinal actions that are particularly helpful against some of the characteristic symptoms of Syndrome X. These flavorful vegetables should be bought and used on a regular basis. Among them are:

- *Garlic,* which lowers cholesterol, triglycerides, blood pressure, and glucose levels
- *Onions and green onions,* which contain many of the same heart-healthy compounds as garlic, but in smaller concentrations
- *Celery,* which contains a compound called 3-n-butyl phthalide, which lowers blood pressure

There's one more thing to say about buying produce: Try to buy organic varieties whenever possible. We certainly don't want to discourage you from buying fresh fruits and vegetables, but commercial produce is sprayed with pesticides, which act like low-dose synthetic estrogens. Many types of produce are also often treated with chemical fungicides (e.g., strawberries) and waxed (e.g., cucumbers). All of these chemicals contribute to a toxic load that taxes liver function, and a stressed-out liver does not do a good job of managing glucose levels.

If the grocery store you typically shop at doesn't carry organic produce, look around at other stores or take a trip to your local natural-food store. Organic produce is becoming increasingly available, and its cost is decreasing. When you cannot buy organic, peel your fruits and vegetables, or use a fruit and vegetable rinse (e.g., OrganiClean, 1-888-VEG-WASH) that contains a food-grade non-ionic surfactant; this can be found in health-food stores.

Shopping in the Meat and Seafood Sections

The main guideline to keep in mind when browsing through the meat and seafood sections is to choose items that are as fresh and unprocessed as possible. The following are a few ways to put this guideline into practice in the supermarket:

- Select fresh, unprocessed chicken and turkey over chicken or turkey that is prebasted, deep basted, or premarinated.
- Choose fresh, unprocessed meats and poultry instead of meats that are smoked and cured.
- Buy fresh fish and seafood over processed forms of these foods, such as fish cakes, crab cakes, and smoked fish.

Red meats, such as beef, are a great source of zinc, a mineral necessary for proper insulin function (which you'll read more about in Chapter 14). Unfortunately, however, most commercial beef has an unhealthy fatty-acid profile because it comes from cattle fattened on grains. Therefore, if you buy beef in supermarkets, it is best to select the leanest cuts available—such as ground round, flank steak, eye of the round, and eye-of-the-round breakfast steaks. A far healthier choice, though, is organic beef from free-range cattle (as well as organic poultry from free-range chickens and turkeys). Organic meats come from animals not treated with steroids and antibiotics; you can find these meats in natural-food stores across the country. In the next few years, many meats will come from animals fed on omega-3-rich mash; these will have a healthier fatty-acid profile than commercial meats today.

Fish spoils more quickly than land-animal meats because of its omega-3 content, so when shopping for seafood, the key is to become savvy about freshness. You can do this in a number of different ways. First, ask the clerk at the seafood counter which fish are the freshest, or ask when different types of fish were delivered.

The clerk's answers to these questions should narrow down your choices. Then look at and smell the fish carefully. Truly fresh fish has a mild and pleasant aroma, like that of a sea breeze. It should not smell "fishy." In addition, the color of whole fish should be uniform, and if you poke the fish with your finger, its flesh should spring right back instead of forming a dent. To prevent the fish from spoiling in your car, you should drive home quickly from the store once you buy fish. If you have a long drive home or if it is a very hot summer day, bring a cooler with blue ice (or get ice from the seafood clerk) and temporarily pack the fish in the cooler to keep it cool on the way home.

Shopping in the Egg, Dairy, Deli, and Perishable-Foods Sections

The refrigerated sections of supermarkets typically contain eggs, dairy products, deli meats, and other perishable foods. You won't need to spend a lot of time in these areas, but carefully selecting foods from these sections can add variety and flavor to the Anti-X style of eating.

Eggs should be tops on your list of foods to buy from these sections. Eggs are a great source of protein with relatively little fat, and numerous studies have found dietary cholesterol such as that found from eggs has little or no effect on blood cholesterol levels. In the diet plans in the next chapter, you'll see that eggs can be eaten often for breakfast, lunch, and snacks. The best types of eggs are those from free-range chickens that wander about and peck at greens, insects, and worms.

Eggs from free-ranging hens have *20* times more omega-3 fatty acids than standard supermarket eggs. These types of eggs are hard to find, but recently another convenient alternative has become available in many supermarkets—eggs from chickens fed an omega-3-rich diet, from either fish meal or flaxseed. These eggs have a much healthier ratio of omega-6 and omega-3 fatty acids, so look for them to gain an extra Anti-X advantage. Brand names of omega-3-enriched eggs include Gold Circle Farms, The Country Hen, Born 3 (as in omega-3), and Pilgrim's Pride's EggPlus.

The best foods to select in the dairy section are—believe it or not—butter, as well as low-fat dairy foods such as nonfat or low-fat cottage cheese and nonfat plain, unsweetened yogurt. Although many people believe otherwise, butter is far healthier for the heart than margarine: Butter, when used in moderation, can therefore be a part of Anti-X eating. (Olive oil, though, should be the preferred dietary fat.) Steer clear of cottage cheese and fruit "snack packs," fruit-flavored yogurt, and fruit-on-the-bottom varieties of yogurt, though. These are almost always loaded with sugar or other sweeteners.

When looking through the cheese, deli, and perishable foods sections, read labels carefully. To choose foods wisely, check the fat and protein content on the label of convenience meat products and cheeses *and* look at their list of ingredients. If the product has a lot of sugar and salt and ingredients that you can't pronounce or spell, much less recognize, the chances are good that the product degrades health more than it promotes health.

Choose products that are as high in protein and as low in fat as possible, and those that have little or no sugar and additives. The best cheeses to select are part-skim mozzarella and feta cheeses, and the best deli meat is low-salt turkey breast. Condiments found in the refrigerator case—such as olives, pesto sauce, and other foods—typically are better for you than foods of this nature found in the inner aisles of the supermarket because they have less salt and additives. Buying perishable foods in the refrigerator case instead of shelf-stable foods in the center of the supermarket is another way of getting fresher foods.

Shopping in the Frozen-Foods Sections

Frozen vegetables are the next best thing to fresh vegetables. At times, they're actually a better choice because they don't go bad quickly. This means you can load up on a wide variety of frozen vegetables and have them in your freezer, ready to cook at a moment's notice.

Nonstarchy vegetable combinations such as Chinese stir-fry vegetables are great ways of getting lots of different types of healthy vegetables. Be sure, though, to look at the list of ingredients and choose those that contain only vegetables. Avoid frozen foods that have seasonings or sauces added to them; they often contain salt, sugar, or partially hydrogenated oils.

Other products worth buying in the frozen-foods sections include unsweetened frozen fruits (be sure that fruits are the only ingredients listed), flash-frozen fish, frozen shrimp, and frozen meats. TV dinners should be avoided; they're loaded with refined grains, sugars, salt, and partially hydrogenated oils, all of which contribute to Syndrome X.

Shopping in the Inner Aisles of the Supermarket

Most of the food products in the inner aisles of the supermarket are made of refined flour, refined sugar, partially hydrogenated oils, or omega-6-rich oils. Therefore, you need to be very selective about the convenience foods you choose. Read labels carefully, and avoid buying any food products that contain flour, partially hydrogenated oils, and hidden forms of sugar, or even natural foods that have a high number of grams of carbohydrates. To keep things easy, we've compiled a quick rundown of the most helpful Anti-X convenience foods to look for when shopping in the inner aisles of your grocery store.

BEVERAGES. The best beverage by far is the only drink that is a nutrient all by itself—water. Bottled water, plain sparkling water, or sparkling water with flavor essences are all healthful choices to buy in supermarkets. Avoid those that contain fruit juices.

HERBAL TEAS, TEA, AND COFFEE. Choose plain, unflavored tea, green tea, and coffee—or better yet, caffeine-free herbal teas. These all can be made cold or hot. As you'll learn in Chapter 16, tea, particularly green tea, is a better choice to begin the day than coffee. Although both black and green tea contain caffeine and are diuretics, they are rich in antioxidant compounds and can lower glucose and triglyceride levels. In contrast, coffee raises glucose levels.

CRACKERS. Look for the lowest-carbohydrate, 100-percent whole-grain rye cracker you can find. The two best choices in many commercial supermarkets are Wasa light rye crispbread (5 grams of carbohydrate per cracker) and Kavli thin crispbread (about 4 grams of carbohydrate per piece). If you can't find these in grocery stores near you, look for them in natural-food or gourmet-food stores.

NUTS AND SEEDS. Look in the baking aisle for raw nuts and seeds, and in the snack food or nut aisle for roasted nuts and seeds, preferably dry-roasted without omega-6-rich oils such as soybean oil, cottonseed oil, or safflower oil. Although many people mistakenly think nuts are not healthy for the heart, numerous studies have found that eating nuts significantly lowers the risk of coronary heart disease. Nuts and seeds are rich in many heart-healthy nutrients, such as magnesium and vitamin E. This makes them convenient snack foods and tasty oatmeal and entree toppers in the Anti-X diet.

CANNED FOODS. Try to find low-salt varieties of canned water-packed tuna, other canned fish, and vegetables such as water chestnuts that typically only come canned. If you can't find low-salt or salt-free varieties, buy the lowest sodium product available, and before you use it, empty the contents of the can into a strainer and rinse it with filtered water. Doing this is particularly important if you have hypertension; it sends much of the excess sodium in these foods down the drain. If you prefer tuna packed in oil over tuna packed in water, avoid tuna packed in soybean oil; instead, go to a specialty store and look for tuna packed in olive oil. If you buy omega-3-rich sardines, choose those that are packed in olive oil over those in soybean oil.

SAUCES. To buy a pasta sauce that fits into the Anti-X diet plan, scan labels to find one without sugar, corn syrup, high-fructose corn syrup, and vegetable oils (such as soybean oil or corn oil) in the list of ingredients. It also should contain no more than 5 grams of sugars per half-cup serving. Classico Tomato-Basil is one commercial item that fits these criteria. A wider selection can be found in natural-food stores.

OILS. Seek out cold-pressed or unrefined extra-virgin olive oil. "Extra-virgin" is important because it means that the oil comes from the first pressing of the olives. Avoid olive oils that are labeled "virgin," "light," or "extra light," because they are more processed and not as healthy.

SALAD DRESSINGS. Look for salad dressings that are made with mono-unsaturated-rich olive oil or canola oil instead of omega-6-rich oils, such as soybean oil. Be sure to avoid dressings that contain sugar or other forms of hidden sugar, and partially hydrogenated oils. The Zeus brand of Greek salad dressings is a particularly good commercial brand.

CONDIMENTS. Read labels and be sure to choose condiments, such as mustard, horseradish, and salsa, that have no sugar added. Other sugar-free condiments, such as capers and olives, also are good to have on hand to use in small amounts on entrees. Salt-free, sugar-free natural peanut butter (made from peanuts alone) is another helpful condiment to buy if you're on a moderate-carbohydrate diet.

SEASONINGS. Buy a wide variety of herbs and spices, and use them liberally to get both flavor and phytonutrients with every shake of the bottle. A few seasonings stand out in their ability to help combat insulin resistance and glucose intolerance; these include cinnamon, cloves, bay leaves, and coriander. (For more information, see Chapter 16.)

GOING THE EXTRA MILE: SHOPPING IN NATURAL-FOOD STORES

We recommend shopping in natural-food supermarkets whenever possible, because they offer more options for Anti-X eating, compared with conventional supermarkets. The clear difference between natural-food supermarkets and conventional supermarkets is that natural-food supermarkets offer a wide selection of organic products—foods not sprayed with pesticides, and meats, eggs, and dairy products from animals not treated with hormones or antibiotics. A cardinal rule for promoting health is to avoid chemicals whenever possible. Shopping in natural-food stores and selecting organic products, therefore, helps enhance health.

It is a big mistake, though, to assume that everything you pick up in a natural-food supermarket is healthful and helpful for preventing insulin resistance. The sugary treats and carbohydrate-based convenience foods in health-food stores may be organic and more nutritious than the convenience foods in typical supermarkets, but they are still going to promote insulin resistance. This means you have to read labels just as carefully as you do in commercial supermarkets, and you must steer clear of high-carbohydrate foods and foods that contain natural, hidden forms of sugar, such as honey and fruit-juice concentrates. You also should continue to follow the most important rule of doing most of your shopping along the perimeter of the store.

What follows is a list of some of the most helpful food items usually sold only in natural-food stores. Many of the following products are good for variety while eating a moderate-carbohydrate diet, but some can be too high in carbohydrates for therapeutic effects when insulin resistance is severe. Those that are safe for people on a low-carbohydrate diet are marked with an asterisk (*).

STEVIA*. This herb has 200–300 times the sweetness of sugar. With negligible calories, it does not raise blood glucose levels like other caloric sweeteners. (See Chapter 16 for more information.) It is typically found in the white extract powder form or as a liquid extract in health-food stores, and it can be used in small amounts to sweeten drinks and foods. Stevia, therefore, is a pretty remarkable product—it is a safe alternative to sugar for diabetics and for everyone with insulin resistance. If your health-food store does not carry stevia, special-order it, or refer to the resources appendix for information on how to order it.

UNREFINED SEA SALT AND HERBAL SALT*. Natural-food stores generally carry a number of healthier alternatives to the refined salt sold in commercial grocery stores. Most regular table salt contains aluminum and sugar; it is refined to remove all naturally occurring minerals besides sodium and chloride; and it is bleached and treated with anticaking agents. It is best, therefore, to avoid table salt when possible. Choose, instead, unrefined sea salt, unrefined rock salt, or herbal salts from the natural-food store. Three products we recommend are Real Salt (an unrefined rock salt), and Bioforce Herbamare and Trocomare herbal salts.

FLAXSEED OIL*. A source of hard-to-find omega-3 fatty acids, unrefined flaxseed oil has a mild nutty or buttery taste. To increase your intake of omega-3 fats, which have Anti-X properties, drizzle small amounts of flaxseed oil on oatmeal or cooked vegetables, mix it with butter for an omega-3-rich spread, or use it by itself or with olive oil in homemade salad dressings. Flaxseed oil needs to be handled carefully: It goes rancid easily, should be kept refrigerated, and should never be heated. Because flaxseed oil is highly perishable, it is found in the refrigerator case of natural-food stores; look for an expiration date on the bottle before buying it.

FLAXSEEDS. Available in packages or in bulk, flaxseeds are tiny brown seeds rich in omega-3 fatty acids. As another way to increase your intake of beneficial omega-3s, try grinding flaxseed and adding it to cooked oatmeal.

NUTS AND SEEDS. Natural-food supermarkets offer a wider selection of raw or lightly toasted nuts and seeds than can be found in traditional supermarkets. Almonds, walnuts, and pumpkin seeds are probably the best nuts to emphasize, but it is good to include small amounts of a variety of nuts and seeds in the diet. The most affordable way to do that is to buy nuts and seeds in the bulk food section of a natural-food supermarket.

PUMPKORN. We recommend Pumpkorn, a snack food sold in health-food stores, because it is a good source of protein and healthy fats, and it is low in carbohydrates. Pumpkorn is made from seasoned dry-roasted pumpkin seeds, which have an almost equal balance of omega-6 fatty acids and omega-3 fatty acids, as well as ample zinc, which helps insulin function more efficiently. Pumpkorn is usually sold in the nut or snack-food aisle of the store. If you can't find it, you can ask the grocery clerk to special-order it for you, or check in the resources appendix on how to contact the manufacturer directly.

NUT BUTTERS. A wide range of nut butters are also offered at natural-food stores. Look for those containing only nuts (i.e., without sugar, honey, salt, or oils). Almond butter, rich in heart-healthy monounsaturated fatty acids, is the nut butter we recommend the most.

GAME MEATS*. Game meats, such as buffalo, venison, and ostrich, are healthy sources of protein to try to find. They are much lower in fat and have much healthier fatty-acid profiles than commercial meats. They are typically found in the frozen-foods sections of natural-food stores (but sometimes in the fresh meat case). They're more expensive than commercial meats, but the price is likely to come down as consumer demand for these meats increases. If your natural-food supermarket does not carry game meats, tell the meat manager of your interest. Natural-food supermarkets will often start offering game meats if they know customers want them.

NORTHWEST NATURAL FISH PRODUCTS. These products, also found in the frozen-foods section of the store, come in three varieties: salmon burgers, halibut burgers, and tuna with pesto medallions. All three are good sources of beneficial omega-3 fatty acids. Heating these fish medallions is a quick and convenient way to increase your omega-3 fatty acid intake if you don't like to cook fish from scratch. Keep in mind, though, that the medallions do contain a wild rice blend, which makes them a moderate-carbohydrate food, not a low-carbohydrate food. This makes them great fast food for many people but not for those with severe insulin-resistance problems.

FROZEN WHOLE-GRAIN WAFFLES. A wide variety of frozen waffles that are free of refined sugar and refined flour are offered in natural-food stores. These whole-grain waffles are much too high in carbohydrates for people with serious insulin resistance, but they can fit into a prevention-type, moderate-carbohydrate diet when used sparingly. We recommend avoiding the waffles made out of whole wheat because wheat is a common trigger food to cravings and overeating for many people. Opt instead for the plain, wheat-free waffles made out of brown rice.

WHOLE-GRAIN BREADS. Also carried in natural-food stores are a wide variety of whole-grain breads. While whole-grain breads typically contain fewer additives and are much more nutritious than commercial breads, they still are a concentrated source of carbohydrates that raise glucose and insulin levels quickly. If you do not have insulin-related problems and want to eat bread from time to time, search for a bread made from whole-grain flours that contains the lowest amount of carbohydrate grams per slice. As we mentioned previously, we recommend avoiding whole wheat because wheat stimulates cravings for carbohydrates in many people. One brand of bread to look for is French Meadow Bakery. It produces tasty whole-grain sourdough breads, including spelt sourdough, a wheat-free bread that contains only 10 grams of carbohydrates per slice, and rye-linseed, a wheat-free bread that contains omega-3-rich flaxseeds.

WHOLE GRAINS. Whole grains such as brown rice, wild rice, and quinoa are nutritious, but they are high in carbohydrates and quickly raise glucose and insulin levels. They should be eaten only in small amounts on a prevention-type, moderate-carbohydrate diet. When buying these products, avoid quick-cooking varieties of these grains; they raise glucose levels higher and more quickly than the regular-cooking varieties. Also try to avoid those with a lot of salt, flavorings, and additives. If you want to add more flavor to plain brown rice, make a pilaf yourself by cooking brown rice in chicken broth.

BROTH. As mentioned previously, broth can be used to add a bit more flavor to cooked grains and to poultry and fish entrees. It is best to avoid commercial brands sold in standard grocery stores because they contain a lot of unhealthy ingredients—hidden forms of sugar, monosodium glutamate, a wide range of additives and preservatives, unhealthy amounts of salt, and sometimes partially hydrogenated oil. Look in health-food stores for products that avoid these ingredients. Be sure, though, to avoid broths that contain honey or fruit-juice concentrates. Two health-food brands we recommend are Pacific Foods of Oregon organic chicken or vegetable broth (found in a box in the soup aisle) and Perfect Addition unsalted beef, chicken, fish, and vegetable stock concentrates (found in the frozen-foods section).

Putting This Chapter into Practice

The key to preventing and reversing Syndrome X is knowing how to navigate through restaurants and supermarkets.

- In restaurants, opt for simple high-protein dishes with sides of vegetables. If you're trying to prevent Syndrome X, you can eat small to moderate amounts of any type of vegetable. If you're trying to reverse Syndrome X, though, choose only nonstarchy vegetables such as salads. Watch out for pastas, breads, and desserts. Most restaurants try hard to accommodate the dietary needs of their customers, so don't hesitate to ask for substitutions.

- In supermarkets, shop the perimeter for fresh foods, such as meats, fish, and vegetables. Minimize your time in the inner aisles, which are dominated by highly processed foods and drinks that promote Syndrome X.

CHAPTER 9

The Anti-X Diets and Recipes

AFTER LEARNING HOW to choose foods wisely in restaurants and supermarkets, you need to combine the foods you have chosen into a tasty diet plan for everyday living. This chapter describes how you can do this with two different menu plans.

Our *Basic Anti-X Diet Plan,* which we describe first, is a moderate-carbohydrate plan primarily designed for the *prevention* of Syndrome X. It is also well suited for people with mild insulin-resistance symptoms, such as those who have one symptom of Syndrome X, people who are slightly overweight, or people who have no overt symptoms but simply don't feel their best.

Our *Anti-X Extra-Healing Diet Plan,* which we also describe in this chapter, is for people who need extra healing to reverse clear-cut symptoms. It will benefit people with adult-onset diabetes, those who have at least two of the indicators of Syndrome X (obesity, hypertension, high cholesterol, or elevated triglycerides), or those who simply want to lose fat and reverse insulin resistance faster than would be possible on the Basic Anti-X Diet Plan. The Anti-X Extra-Healing Diet Plan is very low in carbohydrates, so it is more *therapeutic* than the Basic Anti-X Diet Plan.

Following the menu plans are recipes for both diets; these are simple recipes that even novice cooks should be able to follow. At the end of the chapter are practical tips and shortcuts for making either Anti-X diet plan easier to follow at home.

THE BASIC ANTI-X DIET PLAN: PREVENTIVE AND MILDLY THERAPEUTIC

The Basic Anti-X Diet Plan both prevents and reverses insulin resistance and Syndrome X, but it helps heal only mild cases of these conditions. The Basic Anti-X Diet Plan is right for you if:

- You are healthy and simply want to prevent the development of Syndrome X
- You have low-grade symptoms of glucose intolerance and insulin resistance, such as feeling tired after meals or being a few pounds overweight
- You have only one symptom of Syndrome X, such as elevated blood pressure or elevated cholesterol

As a quick review, the principles of the Basic Anti-X Diet Plan are:

1. Avoid refined carbohydrates—white flour, white rice, white sugar, and other concentrated sweeteners.
2. Eat foods in as natural and fresh a state as possible.
3. Emphasize nonstarchy vegetables as your primary sources of carbohydrates. Eat these freely.
4. Keep your intake of carbohydrate-dense foods moderate. Eat no more than four small servings of whole grains, legumes, starchy vegetables, and fruits per day, with no more than two servings per day of whole grains.
5. Avoid soft drinks, fruit juices, alcohol, and other highly processed drinks.
6. Make an oil change: Eliminate omega-6-rich vegetable oils from your diet, and use cold-pressed, extra-virgin olive oil as your primary oil.
7. Enrich your diet with omega-3 fats whenever you can.
8. Steer clear of trans-fatty acids—found in deep-fried foods, margarine, and foods that contain partially hydrogenated oils.
9. Eat protein—lean meats, fish, poultry, eggs, low-fat cheese or nonfat yogurt, or nuts and nut butters—at every meal and snack.

What follows is a weeklong sample menu plan that incorporates the principles of the Basic Anti-X Diet Plan. Use this menu plan as a resource for meal and snack ideas; you do not necessarily have to follow it to the letter. It simply gives you an idea of some of the things you can eat on an Anti-X eating plan for life.

Keep in mind that the diet is meant to be flexible and changed according to your needs. If you follow the principles of Anti-X eating, you can combine foods in whatever way you like, according to your preferences, allergies/sensitivities, and lifestyle. Learn the diet in the outline form, and make substitutions whenever necessary. The key to successful Anti-X eating is to follow the principles and create a personal program that works for you.

The Basic Anti-X Diet Plan: One-Week Sample Menu

An asterisk (*) indicates that the recipe is included later in this chapter.

Day 1

Breakfast 2 poached eggs on 1 slice of 100-percent
whole-grain rye toast

Lunch ¼ rotisserie-cooked or roasted chicken
(skin removed)
steamed broccoli and cauliflower
green leaf salad with sliced cucumber and radishes,
topped with olive oil vinaigrette dressing

Dinner Filet of Sole Florentine with Spinach and Onions*
½ cup brown rice

Snack 2 part-skim mozzarella cheese sticks
(optional) plum or small peach

Day 2

Breakfast 5 small Turkey Sausage Patties with Fennel
and Sage*
1 wheat-free brown-rice waffle, topped with ½ cup
thawed frozen blueberries and raspberries

Lunch tuna salad with 3 ounces flaked water-packed tuna,
chopped celery, green onion, fresh cilantro, and
1 tablespoon canola mayonnaise on a bed of
lettuce leaves or stuffed in a tomato

Dinner ½ recipe of Roast Cornish Hen with Sage-Thyme
Vegetable Stuffing*
French-cut green beans almondine

| Snack (optional) | 3 celery sticks spread with almond butter |

Day 3

Breakfast	⅔ cup Overnight Oatmeal-Apple-Walnut Muesli*
Lunch	large Greek salad with 3 ounces broiled herb-seasoned chicken strips, romaine lettuce, slivered red onion, sliced cucumber, tomato wedges, 1 teaspoon pumpkin seeds, a few Greek olives, 2 teaspoons crumbled feta cheese with sugar-free olive oil vinaigrette dressing
Dinner	3 small broiled lamb chops seasoned with garlic, oregano, salt, pepper, and lemon juice asparagus steamed artichoke with olive oil/lemon juice/garlic/fresh basil dressing as a dip
Snack (optional)	hard-boiled egg celery sticks

Day 4

Breakfast	2 eggs scrambled with chopped tomatoes, peppers, and onions, topped with sugar-free salsa ½ grapefruit
Lunch	baked fish (any type) basted with garlic butter or caper butter green beans 1 cup strawberries
Dinner	arugula with sugar-free olive oil vinaigrette dressing Greek Chicken with Cinnamon-Spiced Tomato Sauce* 1 cup Baked Spaghetti Squash*
Snack (optional)	⅓ cup pumpkin seeds or Pumpkorn (seasoned dry-roasted pumpkin seeds)

Day 5

| Breakfast | ½ cup nonfat or low-fat cottage cheese
sliver of melon or ½ cup cantaloupe |

Lunch broiled shrimp kabobs, skewered with sliced onion, bell peppers, and mushrooms, brushed with olive oil and herbs, and sprinkled with lemon
½ cup cooked wild rice and brown rice combination or quinoa

Dinner 4 ounces roast turkey breast slices with natural juices
small baked sweet potato or yam with 1½ teaspoons butter and a dash of cinnamon or pumpkin-pie spice
steamed broccoli and cauliflower

Snack (optional) ¼ cup almonds or sunflower seeds

Day 6

Breakfast a few leftover turkey breast slices, sprinkled lightly with unrefined salt, or a few turkey-sausage patties
a few thin part-skim mozzarella cheese slices on 2 Kavli thin rye crispbreads

Lunch broiled organic hamburger, buffalo burger, or turkey burger with lettuce, sliced tomato, and sliced red onion
small baked potato with 1 teaspoon butter and chives

Dinner mixed baby green salad with sugar-free salad dressing
broiled swordfish brushed with olive oil and herbs
green peas with butter

Snack (optional) 2 thin provolone or mozzarella cheese slices wrapped around cooked chilled asparagus spears

Day 7

Breakfast 1 hard-boiled egg
½ cup oatmeal with ½ apple, chopped; a few raisins; 1–2 tablespoons chopped walnuts; and 2 teaspoons ground flaxseeds or flaxseed oil drizzled on top

Lunch chicken fajita with grilled chicken strips, onions, peppers, sugar-free salsa, and guacamole on a corn tortilla

Dinner   Baked Salmon (or Halibut) in Parchment Paper*,
                with assorted vegetables (onion, zucchini,
                broccoli, cauliflower), and olive oil or butter
                and dill seasoning
                ½ cup fresh pineapple cubes

Snack   cucumber slices or red pepper sticks with nonfat
                or low-fat Cottage Cheese–Feta-Dill Spread*

A Note about Beverages

Do not let beverages sabotage the effectiveness of your Anti-X diet. First and foremost, avoid soft drinks, fruit drinks, and fruit beverages, which act like liquid sweets in the body. If, on occasion, you feel you absolutely must have some juice, mix a very small amount of juice with a very big glass of water or sparkling water, and count that as a serving of fruit for the day.

On the Basic Anti-X Diet Plan, most types of alcohol also should be avoided. The research on alcohol is somewhat confusing: Wine may increase insulin sensitivity, but alcohol in general is metabolized by the body as a carbohydrate, depletes nutrients, and can lead to liver dysfunction. For all of these reasons, alcohol is a common contributor to glucose- and insulin-related health problems, particularly in the amounts many people consume it—amounts that make up 5 to 10 percent of total daily calories in the average adult's diet. Our best advice for the prevention of Syndrome X is to avoid alcohol, especially hard liquor, which tends to raise insulin levels. If you are healthy and want a drink on occasion, opt for wine, and count that as a serving of a high-carbohydrate food such as a potato or two servings of fruit.

As a replacement for sugar-sweetened drinks, it may be tempting to consume drinks sweetened with aspartame (NutraSweet or Equal), but we urge you not to: Both NutraSweet and Equal contain sugar disguised as dextrose and/or maltodextrin. Even worse, the safety of aspartame is far from established. More than 75 percent of all nondrug complaints to the FDA concern aspartame, and at least 70 different symptoms and five deaths from its use have been reported. According to physician Russell Blaylock, author of *Excitotoxins: The Taste That Kills* (Santa Fe, New Mexico: Health Press, 1994), the use of aspartame destroys neurons and contributes to the development of brain and nervous-system disorders, such as Alzheimer's disease. Aspartame may not promote insulin resistance, but it should be avoided because it certainly doesn't promote health.

If you do like the taste of a sweet drink from time to time, we recommend familiarizing yourself with the herb stevia (written about in Chapter 15) and using it to make sugar-free versions of drinks, such as lemonade and mint juleps. To make lemonade, for example, mix one-half cup of fresh lemon juice, one-eighth tea-spoon of pure white stevia powder, and four cups of cold water to make four glasses. To learn more about how to purchase stevia or to get books of recipes that use stevia, look in your local health-food store, or see the resources appendix.

Caffeine-containing coffee raises blood glucose levels, especially when consumed in large amounts, so its intake should be kept to a minimum (i.e., no more than two cups per day). Black tea and green tea offer some benefits—they can reduce glucose and triglyc-eride levels (see Chapter 15)—so they're a better choice to start the day than coffee. Teas, however, act as diuretics and contain caf-feine, which can be problematic for many people, so they are best consumed only in moderation.

When all is said and done, the best drink is the one our bodies need on a daily basis—water, preferably filtered or bottled. Sparkling water (plain, with a lemon or lime wedge, or with flavor essences) and caffeine-free herbal teas are other good choices.

Seeing Results on the Basic Anti-X Diet Plan

The length of time it takes to see benefits on the Basic Anti-X Diet Plan varies widely among individuals. Most people, however, start to see some positive changes in their health—anything from expe-riencing more energy or fewer food cravings to having a flatter tummy—within just a week or two of eating the Anti-X way. It often takes longer, however, to see decreases in blood pressure and cho-lesterol.

Glucose tolerance can be improved within a single day, so many people begin to feel more alert and energetic and less moody fairly quickly. It's also common to experience some initial, quick weight loss of a few pounds, but this usually slows down after a week or two, because it's mostly water weight. Then, a slow but steady loss of fat—say, a pound or two a week—often occurs. Again, individual responses vary, so if this doesn't occur with you, don't become con-cerned. However, if you don't experience any signs of fat loss (such as pants fitting better) within a month of following the Basic Anti-X

Diet Plan, switch to the more therapeutic Anti-X Extra-Healing Diet Plan to jump-start the body's ability to burn fat.

Once you have gotten the results you're looking for on the Basic Anti-X Diet Plan, you shouldn't totally go off the diet. If you do, you'll end up redeveloping the same problems that have bothered you. To make this program work for you for the long term, it's important to learn to modify the diet so that it becomes a flexible eating plan that you can follow for the rest of your life.

Modifying the Basic Anti-X Diet Plan to Make It a Diet for Life

Once you are in good health, feel well, and are at your desired weight for several months, you can occasionally sidestep the principles of the Anti-X diet and eat a high-carbohydrate meal. This is the way to make the Basic Anti-X Diet Plan fit into your lifestyle so you can enjoy vegetarian food, a whole-grain pasta dish, an alcoholic drink, or a dessert with friends one evening instead of feeling like a party pooper who has to go against the grain all the time.

If you are like most people who follow the Anti-X diet, you may very well find that you don't feel as well after you eat a high-carbohydrate meal as you do when you eat according to the principles of the Anti-X diet. Listen to these signals: They are your body's way of telling you to stick to the Anti-X diet to continue looking and feeling your best.

Holidays and vacations are times when most of us indulge in too many carbohydrates, and it is important not to let such situations completely derail you from the Anti-X diet. On holidays and vacations, therefore, pay special attention to how you feel. If you start to feel less mentally sharp or more physically sluggish, if your waist starts to feel bloated, if your weight creeps up, or if you have trouble putting on your favorite pair of pants, take these as clear warnings that you need to take corrective action before things go further downhill: Simply avoid all high-carbohydrate foods and get back to lean animal protein and lots of nonstarchy veggies. Within a few days, you should be back to feeling your healthy and trim self.

The key to transforming the Basic Anti-X Diet Plan into a protective diet for life is recognizing that you may want to splurge with a high-carbohydrate meal from time to time, but afterward, you must get right back on the Basic Anti-X Diet Plan to prevent Syndrome X and all the complications that accompany this condition. To avoid going down the same path of insulin-related health problems later in life that so many North Americans do, do not stray too much from the diet for too long.

THE ANTI-X EXTRA-HEALING DIET PLAN: HIGHLY THERAPEUTIC, FOR THOSE WITH SEVERE INSULIN RESISTANCE

The Anti-X Extra-Healing Diet Plan stimulates quicker and more aggressive reversal of insulin resistance. The Anti-X Extra-Healing Diet Plan is right for you if:

- You have at least two of the indicators of Syndrome X (obesity, hypertension, high cholesterol, or elevated triglycerides)
- You have tried the Basic Anti-X Diet Plan and have been unable to get the weight loss results or improvements in blood pressure, cholesterol, or triglycerides that you want
- You have adult-onset diabetes

The principles of the Anti-X Extra-Healing Diet Plan are similar to the principles of the Basic Anti-X Diet Plan, except for two key differences. These differences are as follows:

1. Eat nonstarchy vegetables as your *main* sources of carbohydrates. (The Anti-X Extra-Healing Diet Plan also provides very limited quantities of carbohydrates in the form of low-carbohydrate rye crackers, nuts and seeds, and low-fat cheeses and cottage cheese.) Eat nonstarchy vegetables freely, but completely eliminate starchy vegetables, legumes, whole grains, and fruits from your diet.

2. To satisfy your appetite, eat more lean, protein-rich meats and healthy fats—especially omega-3 fatty acids found in fatty fish, flaxseed oil, and pumpkin seeds, and monounsaturated fatty acids found in olive oil, pesto sauce, and such nuts as almonds and macadamias. Do not be afraid to eat protein and fat; they will not lead to weight gain, as long as you do not overdo carbohydrates. Keep in mind that if you crave carbohydrates, you are probably not eating enough protein.

The Anti-X Extra-Healing Diet Plan is safe for virtually everyone, but it does come with just a few cautions: It should not be followed by people about to undergo surgery or pregnant women—and probably not by those with liver or kidney problems, unless under the supervision of a health professional. Those with insulin-dependent diabetes or type 2 diabetes on medications should work with their doctors while following the diet because medication dosages may have to be adjusted.

What follows is a recommendation for implementing the principles of the Anti-X Extra-Healing Diet Plan in a weeklong menu. Remember, though, to personalize the menu according to your needs, preferences, and allergies/sensitivities. If you do not like a meat or a nonstarchy vegetable listed on the menu, make a substitution with something similar. Just make sure to continue to follow the basic principles outlined previously.

The Anti-X Extra-Healing Diet Plan: One-Week Sample Menu

Day 1

Breakfast	3 eggs scrambled in olive oil with chopped tomatoes, peppers, and onions, topped with sugar-free salsa, if desired
Lunch	½ rotisserie-cooked or roasted chicken (skin removed) steamed broccoli and cauliflower mixed baby green salad with red pepper slices topped with vinegar and olive oil dressing or other sugar-free salad dressing
Dinner	Filet of Sole Florentine*, with spinach, onions, and lemon juice
Snack (optional)	a few olives a few turkey slices dabbed with pesto sauce or mustard

Day 2

Breakfast	5 small Turkey Sausage Patties with Fennel and Sage* 1 Kavli thin rye crispbread, spread with almond butter or sugar-free peanut butter
Lunch	tuna salad with 6 ounces canned, flaked tuna, mixed with minced green onion, celery, and fresh cilantro, and 1 tablespoon canola mayonnaise served on top of a bed of green lettuce leaves

Dinner	roast Cornish hen brushed with olive oil and herbs green beans sautéed greens of any type, with garlic in olive oil

Snack (optional)   a few tablespoons pumpkin seeds or Pumpkorn

Day 3

Breakfast   2 hard-boiled eggs sprinkled lightly with herbal salt
5 celery sticks filled with Cottage Cheese–Feta-Chive
   Spread*

Lunch   large Greek salad with 4 ounces of broiled
   herb-seasoned chicken strips, with romaine
   lettuce, slivered red onion, sliced cucumber,
   tomato wedges, 1 teaspoon pumpkin seeds, a few
   Greek olives, 2 teaspoons crumbled feta cheese
   with sugar-free olive oil vinaigrette dressing

Dinner   3 small broiled lamb chops with garlic, oregano,
   and lemon juice
grilled sliced zucchini and eggplant, brushed with
   olive oil and seasoned with herbs

Snack (optional)   a handful of almonds

Day 4

Breakfast   small breakfast steak quick-seared in olive oil with
   sliced mushrooms, garlic, and French-cut green
   beans

Lunch   2 swordfish kabobs, skewered with onion pieces,
   green and red pepper chunks, and mushrooms,
   seasoned with herbs and brushed with olive oil
   and a squeeze of lemon

Dinner   chicken stir fry with chicken, Chinese cabbage,
   bean sprouts, ginger, garlic, green onions, and a
   few water chestnuts, cooked in unrefined sesame
   oil and topped with a teaspoon of toasted sesame
   seeds and a dash of wheat-free tamari soy sauce

Snack (optional)   hard-boiled egg or Pesto-Deviled Egg*

Day 5

Breakfast	leftover chicken stir fry
Lunch	6 cooked shrimp, chilled, served with dipping sauce of pesto mixed with lemon juice 4 tomato slices topped with thin mozzarella cheese slices and fresh basil, drizzled with olive oil vinaigrette salad dressing
Dinner	4 ounces roast turkey breast slices with natural juices double serving of steamed broccoli and cauliflower with butter
Snack (optional)	5 macadamia nuts

Day 6

Breakfast	4 turkey breast slices or turkey sausage patties 1 Kavli thin rye crispbread, topped with 1 thin slice low-fat cheese
Lunch	broiled organic hamburger, buffalo burger, or turkey burger with lettuce, sliced tomato, and sliced red onion Chilled Cucumber–Red Onion Salad* or ½ cup sauerkraut
Dinner	trout almondine steamed asparagus with butter red leaf and radicchio salad with sugar-free salad dressing
Snack (optional)	cucumber sticks or red pepper slices with Cottage Cheese–Feta-Dill Spread*

Day 7

Breakfast	3 eggs scrambled in olive oil with spinach, green onions, a few crumbles of feta cheese and dill seasoning, topped with a dab of pesto sauce after cooking
Lunch	roast duck or any type of lean meat red cabbage and onions sautéed in olive oil

Dinner   Baked Salmon (or Halibut) in Parchment Paper*,
                with zucchini, broccoli, cauliflower, onion, olive
                oil, butter, and dill

Snack   a few turkey or chicken breast slices
(optional)   a few celery sticks

Sugar-Free Beverages to Choose From
(in order from best to worst)

Filtered or bottled water, plain or with a lemon wedge; sparkling
mineral water; caffeine-free herbal teas; plain, unsweetened, unflavored green or black tea; plain coffee without sugar (no more than
two cups per day)

Seeing Results on the Anti-X Extra-Healing Diet Plan

The Anti-X Extra-Healing Diet Plan is more therapeutic than the
Basic Anti-X Diet Plan, so weight loss and improvements in blood
pressure, cholesterol, and triglycerides (as well as glucose and insulin levels) often begin to occur quickly. If you're taking medication
to control any of these conditions, it's best to work with a physician
who can monitor these indicators and work with you to adjust the
medication and gradually wean yourself off it, as appropriate.

Keep in mind, though, that Syndrome X is an insidious condition that develops over time. Therefore, it can't be cured overnight.
Be patient and realize that it took a while to develop this condition,
so it also will take a while—often six months or so—for the body to
reverse this condition. The length of time for healing is very individual, but as a general rule, the longer you've had symptoms of
Syndrome X, the longer it usually takes to totally reverse and clear
these symptoms.

Moving from the Anti-X Extra-Healing Diet Plan
to the Basic Anti-X Diet Plan

Once you have largely reversed severe insulin resistance, you can
and should make a gradual transition from the Anti-X Extra-
Healing Diet Plan to the Basic Anti-X Diet Plan. The indicators
that can tell you that you are ready to make the transition from the

stronger corrective action of the Anti-X Extra-Healing Diet Plan to the Basic Anti-X Diet Plan are as follows:

- When you have normalized your blood pressure, blood cholesterol, or blood triglyceride readings and these values have remained in healthy ranges for two months
- When you no longer have two or more strong indicators of Syndrome X (overweight, high triglycerides, high cholesterol, and high blood pressure)
- When you have normalized your blood glucose levels and have (with your doctor's permission) eliminated any antidiabetic medicines you may have been taking to lower glucose levels
- When you have reached your ideal weight or come within five pounds of your ideal weight after previously trying the Basic Anti-X Diet Plan without successfully losing weight

When these signs are favorable, you can begin making the transition from the more carbohydrate-restricted diet to the moderate-carbohydrate diet by adding to your diet one serving each day of a carbohydrate food other than nonstarchy vegetables. We suggest adding fruit back first because it is generally low in carbohydrates and low on the glycemic index, and it is more in keeping with our genetic heritage than are other types of carbohydrates, such as grains and legumes. Some of the best fruits to try adding back are 1 cup strawberries, raspberries, or blueberries; half a grapefruit; or an apple.

If you eat an additional serving of fruit each day for one week and don't gain weight or feel bloated or notice any other adverse symptoms, keep going. Add another serving of a high-carbohydrate food such as starchy vegetables, legumes, or whole grains each day for a week. Each week for the next four weeks, keep adding one more serving of nutritious carbohydrates such as fruits, starchy vegetables, legumes, and whole grains to your diet until you reach the guidelines for the Basic Anti-X Diet Plan—four servings total per day of these high-carbohydrate foods, with no more than two servings from whole grains. (We suggest adding whole wheat back last because it is a common trigger food to cravings and overeating for many people.)

If, in the process of adding back another serving of carbohydrates, you find yourself gaining weight, craving carbohydrates, or not feeling well in other ways, go back to the level of carbohydrates you were able to eat without having problems. Everyone has a different amount of carbohydrates he or she thrives on. By participating in this trial-and-error process, you can design a personalized diet that contains the ideal amount of carbohydrates for you. If you continue adding back servings of carbohydrates without any problems until you reach the diet that's the Basic Anti-X Diet Plan, simply follow it and learn how to modify it so you can live with it for the rest of your life.

RECIPES

The following are tasty, easy recipes of entrees, side dishes, and snacks listed in the menu plans of one or both Anti-X diet plans. All recipes and both meal plans were developed by nutritionist Melissa Diane Smith.

Filet of Sole Florentine

> 4 cups baby spinach leaves
> 1 tablespoon extra-virgin olive oil
> 1 cup finely chopped onions
> grated nutmeg
> 1 pound sole, flounder, or other mild-tasting fish fillets
> 1 teaspoon olive oil
> the fresh juice of 1 medium to large lemon
> 1–2 tablespoons dill weed or Spice Hunter Deliciously Dill
>   seasoning (a combination of dill weed, onion flakes, lemon
>   peel, and chives)

Wash the spinach well, then steam it for 3 minutes or until wilted. Place 1 tablespoon oil and onions in a frying pan. Sauté the onions until barely soft, then add the spinach, sprinkle with nutmeg, and stir. Arrange the fish in a single layer over the spinach. Drizzle lightly with lemon juice and 1 teaspoon oil, and sprinkle with seasoning.

Cover the pan, cook on medium-low heat, and check after 5 to 7 minutes. (Scoop underneath the fish and spinach mixture once, to make sure it isn't drying out or burning.) The fish is done when it's milky in color and flakes easily with a fork. Sprinkle with extra lemon juice at the table, if desired. Serves 2 to 3.

Turkey Sausage Patties with Fennel and Sage

1 pound lean, organic, ground turkey
4–7 garlic cloves, crushed and pressed
1 teaspoon rubbed sage
1 teaspoon ground fennel
¼ teaspoon fennel seeds (optional)
unrefined, natural sea salt to taste (optional)

Preheat an oven to 350 degrees. Mix all the ingredients, shape the meat mixture into 2-inch-round sausage patties, and place in a baking pan to bake. After baking about 20 minutes, pour off the excess grease from the pan, and dab the patties lightly with a paper towel. Return the pan to the oven for 5 more minutes, or until the patties are done, with no pink coloring in the center. Add unrefined sea salt, to taste, at the table, if desired. Serves 3 to 4.

Roast Cornish Hen with Sage-Thyme Vegetable Stuffing

1 Cornish hen, cut in half
2 teaspoons unrefined, extra-virgin olive oil
4 shallots, diced
1 carrot, diced
1 stalk celery, diced
3 cloves garlic, minced
1 teaspoon sage
½ teaspoon ground thyme
1½ teaspoons chicken broth or water
1 tablespoon chopped fresh chives (optional)

In a large bowl, toss the diced vegetables with the olive oil and herbs, then add the hen halves and rub the mixture over the hens to coat them with the olive oil and herbs. Mix well, so everything is moist. Pour the chicken broth or water in the bottom of a baking pan, then place the vegetable mixture in two separate mounds in the pan. Top each mound with half of a Cornish hen, folding as much of the vegetable mixture as possible under the hens. Bake at 350 degrees for 1 hour. Before serving, top with chopped chives, if desired. Serves 2.

Overnight Oatmeal-Apple-Walnut Muesli

1 cup nonfat plain yogurt
1 cup raw regular (slow-cooking) oats
⅓ cup water
¼ cup raisins
1 small or ½ large Granny Smith or other apple, chopped
½ teaspoon pumpkin-pie spice
½ teaspoon ground cinnamon
⅓ cup chopped walnuts
1½ tablespoons more water

The night before you want to have the muesli, mix together the yogurt, water, and oats in a large bowl, then add the raisins, apple, and spices, and mix everything thoroughly. Cover the mixing bowl with a lid, and refrigerate it overnight. The next morning, add 1½ tablespoons more water, and stir; add slightly more water, as needed, to create a creamy, nonstiff texture. Stir in the walnuts, add a sprinkling more cinnamon if desired, and serve. Serves 3.

Greek Chicken with Cinnamon-Spiced Tomato Sauce

4 large skinless chicken breast halves with ribs
1 tablespoon plus 2 teaspoons extra-virgin olive oil, divided
1 medium yellow onion, chopped
3 garlic cloves, crushed and minced
3 cups sugar-free pasta sauce
1½ teaspoons ground cinnamon
2 bay leaves
feta cheese

Preheat an oven to 350 degrees. Brown the chicken breast pieces on both sides in 1 tablespoon olive oil, then remove them from the cooking pan, and set them aside. Pour the excess grease out, and add the remaining 2 teaspoons olive oil to the pan. Sauté the chopped onion a few minutes until the pieces turn translucent, then add the minced garlic and sauté a minute or so more. Add the onion, garlic, and cinnamon to the pasta sauce, and mix well. Put chicken in a baking dish, and pour the pasta sauce mixture over it. Insert the bay leaves.

Bake the chicken, covered, for 45 minutes, then remove the cover and spoon some sauce on top of the chicken. Bake the chicken 15 to 20 minutes more, until the chicken is done in the center. Remove the bay leaves and serve the chicken and sauce on top of Baked Spaghetti Squash*, and sprinkle each serving with a few teaspoons of crumbled feta cheese. Serves 4.

Baked Spaghetti Squash

As the name implies, spaghetti squash is a nutrient- and fiber-rich substitute for spaghetti. Most people aren't familiar with how to make it, but the instructions are actually quite easy.

1 spaghetti squash

Preheat an oven to 375 degrees. With a long-tined fork, make deep pierces into the skin of the squash in several places and place it in a baking dish or on top of a piece of aluminum foil. Bake the squash for about 30 minutes, or until the skin is soft to the touch. Let the squash cool for 10 minutes, then cut it in half lengthwise, and use a spoon to remove the seeds and strings from the center of the squash. Then use two forks to fluff up the flesh of the squash until you have spaghetti-like strands. Transfer the strands to serving plates, and top with sauce. Serves 4.

Baked Salmon (or Halibut) with Vegetables in Parchment Paper

2 fresh salmon or halibut fillets (about ⅔ to ¾ pound total)
1 zucchini, sliced into ¼-inch rounds
1 small onion, cut into eighths
florets from 1 small stalk broccoli
½ cup chopped florets of cauliflower
1 tablespoon melted butter
1 tablespoon extra-virgin olive oil
dill, flaked onion, and parsley
1 cup water or vegetable broth
2 large sheets unbleached parchment paper

Preheat an oven to 375 degrees. Place a large sheet of parchment paper on a baking dish, and place the fish fillets on the paper. Sprinkle the vegetable pieces on both sides of the fish fillets. Sprinkle seasonings liberally over the entire dish, drizzle a combination of olive oil and melted butter over the fish, then pour the water or broth into the pan. Pull off another large sheet of parchment paper, place it over the fish and vegetables, and roll the edges of the two pieces of parchment paper together to seal the fish and vegetables inside. Bake for about 25 minutes, until the fish is done and flakes easily with a fork. Serves 2.

Cottage Cheese–Feta-Chive Spread

½ cup nonfat or low-fat cottage cheese
1 tablespoon chopped fresh chives
2 teaspoons crumbled feta cheese (optional)
⅛ teaspoon garlic powder (optional)
¼ teaspoon dried Mediterranean oregano leaves
    (optional)

Place ingredients in a bowl, and mash with a potato masher. For best taste, refrigerate for at least several hours. Serves 1 to 2. This recipe can easily be doubled or tripled to serve more people.

Variation. To make Cottage Cheese–Feta-Dill Spread, stir 1 tablespoon chopped fresh dill along with feta cheese into cottage cheese, and chill for several hours or even a day, to allow the fresh dill to impart its flavor. Experiment with other herb combinations—such as sugar-free, salt-free onion dip mixes—to make variations to suit your taste.

Pesto-Deviled Egg

1 hard-boiled egg
1–2 teaspoons pesto sauce (to taste)

Peel a hard-boiled egg, and cut it in half lengthwise. Remove the yolk, and transfer it to a small bowl. Use the back of a spoon to mash the yolk, then add the pesto, and mix well. Transfer the egg-pesto mixture back into the cooked egg-white halves, and serve.

Chilled Cucumber–Red Onion Salad

   1 large cucumber
   ⅛ to ¼ medium red onion, thinly sliced (to your taste)
   1 plum tomato, thinly sliced, or 3–4 cherry tomatoes, halved
      (optional)
   ¼ cup Zeus Greek salad dressing or other sugar-free olive-oil
      vinaigrette salad dressing
   1 tablespoon chopped fresh dill or mint

   Peel the cucumbers, if desired, and thinly slice them. Place the slices in a salad bowl, along with the red onion and tomato. Sprinkle the dill or mint over the salad, then drizzle with the salad dressing and toss well. Cover the bowl, and chill in the refrigerator for several hours for best taste. Serves 2. Recipe can be doubled or tripled.

TIPS FOR FOLLOWING THE ANTI-X DIET AT HOME

The Anti-X diet probably differs from the way you've been eating, and it can be hard to change long-standing habits, unless you prepare yourself mentally and practically speaking for the changes. To help make the diet as easy as possible to follow, it is important to teach yourself some new tricks—in other words, you should take the time to rethink old ideas about food and learn some new food-preparation and eating habits. Here are several practical suggestions:

   ■ Make sure to have some protein for breakfast every morning. Keep in mind that breakfast is the break to the long stretch of time—quite literally, the fast—that you have experienced from dinner to morning. It is vital that you get protein in the morning to stabilize your blood sugar and to prevent cravings for quick-fix carbohydrates later on in the day. Do not get into the rut, though, of thinking that you can only start the day eating traditional breakfast foods such as eggs. If you do, you will get bored fast. Instead, be creative with your choices, and break through the bonds of conventional fare. Breakfast should be any protein-rich meal that gets you off to a good, energetic start. Lunch or dinner foods or leftovers can make great morning meals.
   ■ Plan ahead. If you wait to think about what to eat until you're starved, the chances are that you will sabotage your diet quickly by grabbing ready-to-eat carbohydrate-based convenience foods for

quick energy. These are exactly the foods you need to avoid for success in preventing and reversing Syndrome X. To prevent this from happening, keep your refrigerator and freezer well stocked with protein-rich eggs, poultry, lean meats, and fish, and make sure to set aside enough time in your schedule to prepare these foods.

■ Keep meals simple. Meal preparation does not have to be a time-consuming, elaborate production. To the contrary, the simpler the preparation of a meal, the better it usually is for both you and your body. It doesn't require much time, for example, to broil a piece of fish or a lamb chop and to steam some vegetables—and even slice up some fruit for dessert.

■ Make more food than you plan to eat in one sitting, to create leftovers for snacks or quick meals later in the week. For example, try roasting a chicken or turkey or a beef or lamb roast on the weekend, then cut off the fat and skin, and store the extra sliced meat in your fridge. Later in the week, when you need a snack, grab a few pieces of meat for a quick, convenient, protein pick-me-up. When you come home late from work one night and are too busy to cook a meal from scratch, reheat the meat in broth or a light tomato sauce, and cook up some vegetables for a superquick, balanced meal. You can also slice the meat into strips and sprinkle the strips on top of a large salad for a great lunch or light dinner. Purposely making leftovers—and using them creatively—makes it much easier to follow the diet.

■ Look for other shortcuts to healthy meal preparation, especially when you are busy and under stress. Have the meat-counter clerk cut meat up for you for quick stir-fries or kabobs. Select one of a variety of innovative, prepackaged, prewashed salad mixes in the cold section of the produce department. If you pick up one of these and toss some leftover meat on it, you have fast food at its best. Many grocery stores also have salad bars; you can select a variety of nonstarchy vegetables to make a custom-designed salad, or you can avoid the salad greens and just pick up prechopped vegetables to snack on or steam or stir-fry. This survival strategy really pays off when you just feel too tired to chop a lot of different types of vegetables at the end of a long day. It is also particularly helpful when you are cooking for one. Buying prechopped vegetables is a great shortcut to getting a lot of different veggies in your diet without a lot of fuss.

■ Keep sweets and other highly processed snack foods out of the house, to avoid tempting yourself. Instead, stock healthful, easy-to-grab, sugar-free foods that are ready and waiting for snack attacks. Protein-rich foods to have in your fridge include hard-boiled eggs, cooked meats, cans of low-sodium tuna, and mozzarella cheese sticks; you should also keep on hand veggie sticks and fruits, low-carbohydrate companions to the protein foods. Although they're higher in fat than protein, nuts and Pumpkorn are nutrient-powerhouse foods that work well as snacks—at home or away from home.

■ Be patient with yourself when making the transition from your old way of eating to your new way of eating. It usually takes time to modify long-standing cooking and eating habits, so if you're not instantly perfect about cooking and eating the Anti-X way, don't get frustrated and give up. Have compassion for yourself, and remember that you're only human. Virtually all of us fall off the wagon of Anti-X eating from time to time, but the important thing is whether we get back on the wagon after a momentary transgression or we stay off.

To make sure you are one of those people who gets back on and stays on, keep reminding yourself of the need for these dietary changes. You might want to post a note up on your fridge, saying something like, "Eating my old way got me into my health problems. Eating my new way will get me out." Continue to remember that Syndrome X is a nutritional disease: Bad nutrition is one of the main causes; good nutrition is one of the main cures.

Putting This Chapter into Practice

Our Basic Anti-X Diet Plan and Anti-X Extra-Healing Diet Plan are designed for the needs of two different types of people.

- The Basic Anti-X Diet Plan is a moderate-protein, moderate-carbohydrate diet primarily designed to prevent Syndrome X. However, it can also reverse mild symptoms of insulin resistance and Syndrome X.

- The Anti-X Extra-Healing Diet Plan is a higher-protein, low-carbohydrate diet designed for reversing more serious symptoms of Syndrome X and adult-onset diabetes. It differs from many other protein-rich diets because it emphasizes fowl, fish, and healthy fats, while deemphasizing beef, pork, and unhealthy fats.

CHAPTER 10

A Rational Approach
to Fitness and
Physical Activity

Physical activity is the second part of the one-two punch needed to help both prevent and reverse overweight, insulin resistance, and Syndrome X. Virtually all of us have heard about the benefits of exercise, but most of us think that if we cannot run, take aerobics, or do some other structured exercise (that we force ourselves to engage in several times a week), we are not going to get the benefits of exercise. We give up because we think it has to be all or nothing.

This assumption simply isn't true. Increasing physical activity just a little offers dramatic health benefits. In addition, physical activity does not have to mean structured exercise. It can be as simple as gardening, taking the stairs instead of the elevator, dancing with your spouse, or walking your dog several times a week. Physical activity can be so much fun and so easy to incorporate into your lifestyle that you won't even consider it exercise. Yet by combining moderate physical activity with the Anti-X diet, you will create a formidable defense that will help hold overweight and Syndrome X at bay throughout your lifetime.

COMPARING PHYSICAL ACTIVITY
THEN AND NOW

As we explained in Chapter 5, the activity level of human lifestyles has changed as dramatically as the types of food eaten. Our Paleolithic ancestors trekked long distances on foot in search of food, picked and gathered plant foods by hand, hauled the food they gathered back to others, and ran in short bursts for survival—both to hunt animals and to run away from animals. The type of physical activity our distant ancestors engaged in was regular and continuous, and it mostly involved walking.

Today the most exercise many North Americans get is walking briefly to and from the car and giving their thumbs a workout by channel-surfing with the TV remote control.

On the other side of the coin are a much smaller group of people who do exercise. They generally fall into several categories:

- Weekend warriors, who don't exercise during the week but exercise like crazy (usually in sports) on the weekends
- Reluctant "model" exercisers, who grudgingly go to exercise class and follow the generally recommended guidelines to participate in cardiovascular aerobic exercise for at least 30 minutes three or more times a week;
- Runners, weight-lifters, and other athletes who engage in vigorous exercise or extreme weight-bearing exercise several times a week
- People who walk a lot and are moderately physically active in other ways throughout the day

Which of these types of people are physically active in a way most in keeping with the way our Paleolithic ancestors were active? The last group, by a long shot. Physical activity in the form of walking and engaging in such activities as gardening may not seem like exercise—it hasn't been hyped as such—but it is. What's more, this type of physical activity is much better for you in the long run than the type of exercise most people think of as exercise.

Let's take a quick look at the trouble with the other three types of exercise. Weekend warriors run into several problems. They don't exercise at all during most of the week, so their muscles and cardiovascular system are generally out of shape. Then, when they exercise for several hours in a row on the weekends, the exercise they engage in becomes a stress to their systems, and they often end up with sore muscles for a couple of days. Because weekend warriors are generally out of shape, they are also more prone to injury. Even worse, their hearts are as out of shape as their other muscles. Overdoing exercise on the weekend, therefore, stresses the cardiovascular system and can lead to greater likelihood of a heart attack.

Reluctant "model" exercisers are usually very health-conscious people who are trying hard to do the right thing—to engage in aerobic exercise at least three times a week, as advocated by many exercise physiologists and health organizations. (They are often the same people who follow the widely recommended low-fat, high-carbohydrate diet and can't understand why they keep gaining weight even though they're doing everything "right.") The trouble is they typically dislike the exercise they do, and they pass up other fun activities to drag themselves to exercise class. Dislike of exercise leads to two problems. First, anytime we dislike something, we generally resent it and usually rebel against it. Dropout rates from exercise classes are high, and if we drop out, we often get disgusted with ourselves and decide not to exercise at all because it's such a drag. Second, even if we somehow ignore our feelings and force ourselves to go to class, we don't get as many benefits as we should from exercise because we don't experience joy in what we're doing.

People who engage in vigorous exercise or extreme weight-bearing exercise several times a week experience a high risk of injuries. That's because these types of exercise go against our ancestral nature. Humans didn't evolve to run on pavement for miles at a time day after day, but to walk throughout the day. They also didn't evolve to bench-press 150 or more pounds a few times in a row, but to carry lighter loads—young children or 10–30 pounds of food—for longer stretches of time. Running or weight-lifting may be appropriate for some people, but not for all people. The more we can replicate the type of moderate, continuous activity our ancestors did, the better off we will be. In addition, the more we'll enjoy physical activity and want to continue it on a regular basis.

THE BENEFITS OF REGULAR EXERCISE

The benefits of regular exercise are many and well-established. Such exercise

- Helps the body burn calories to control or lose weight
- Builds muscle and increases muscle strength
- Lowers body fat
- Increases insulin sensitivity (or receptivity) in normal subjects, the insulin-resistant children of diabetic parents, and diabetics
- Boosts immunity, helping the body to fend off illness and disease

- Helps build bone density in people under 30 and slows bone loss in older people
- Boosts optimism and feelings of well-being
- Significantly reduces stress, anxiety, and depression
- Improves sleep, concentration, and academic performance
- Lowers blood glucose, cholesterol, and triglyceride levels
- Reduces blood pressure
- Significantly reduces the risk of cardiovascular disease, Type 2 diabetes, and other diseases

THE NEWFOUND BENEFITS OF MODERATE PHYSICAL ACTIVITY

The health benefits of regular exercise are well-established. Several studies in the 1990s, though, showed that integrating health-enhancing activities into our daily lives is as effective as regular structured exercise—and easier to keep up.

In one study, researchers at the Cooper Institute for Aerobics Research in Dallas randomly divided 235 healthy but sedentary men and women ages 35–60 years into two groups. One group spent 20–60 minutes vigorously exercising—swimming or biking, for example—up to five days a week. The other group incorporated a total of 30 minutes a day of moderate-intensity lifestyle activities such as walking, climbing stairs, and around-the-house chores such as vacuuming and leaf raking. After six months and again after two years, both groups showed significant improvements in cardiorespiratory fitness, blood pressure, and body-fat percentage. There were no significant differences in the degree of improvement between the two groups.

In another study, 40 obese women ages 21–60 years were randomly divided into structured- and lifestyle-activity groups similar to those used in the Dallas study. All participants were asked to adhere to a calorie-restricted diet. After just four months, both groups showed significant and comparable improvement in fat loss, reduced LDL (bad) cholesterol, lowered blood pressure, and increased oxygen intake (a measure of heart-lung fitness). Furthermore, after one year, the lifestyle group had regained less weight than the structured group had.

Increasing physical activity even moderately also helps prevent adult-onset diabetes. One retrospective study that tracked the lifestyle habits and health status of men during a 14-year period found that men who were the most sedentary faced twice the risk of diabetes as men who were the most active. The protective effect of physical activity is strongest in persons at the highest risk for adult-onset diabetes—such as those who are overweight, who have a history of hypertension, or who have parents who are diabetic.

Participating in nonintense physical activity a little more often also improves insulin sensitivity in ways similar to that of vigorous exercise. This means that if you increase simple activities such as walking and doing household chores, you help insulin work more efficiently so that prediabetes conditions such as insulin resistance and Syndrome X won't develop.

HOW PHYSICAL ACTIVITY HELPS PREVENT AND REVERSE INSULIN RESISTANCE

Physical activity is effective medicine against insulin resistance, overweight, Syndrome X, and diabetes because it builds muscle, increases the percentage of muscle in the body, and decreases body fat. Muscle cells are more responsive than fat cells when it comes to dealing with insulin and glucose, and conditioned muscles are more responsive to insulin and glucose than are unconditioned muscles. This means that the more regularly you move your muscles throughout your body, the more you build them up. The more you build up your muscles, the more you enhance your body's sensitivity to insulin, and the more efficiently insulin works to keep glucose levels in normal ranges in your body.

Studies show that physically fit people secrete less insulin after being given carbohydrates than do people who are out of shape. In other words, stepping up physical activity even a little helps the body process carbohydrates more efficiently. Physical activity, therefore, is a terrific counterpart to the Anti-X diet: Even when you aren't always perfect on the diet, physical activity pinch-hits and helps to prevent the development of insulin resistance. Combining moderate physical activity and the Anti-X diet works best of course, because this is a modern-day version of the program that prevented insulin resistance in our Paleolithic ancestors.

UNDERSTANDING PHYSICAL ACTIVITY IN NEW TERMS

You can take heart if you are one of many people who do not like the type of exercise typically recommended by the experts. Ideally, physical activity should be incorporated often throughout the day, and it should be fun.

A new definition of beneficial physical activity, in fact, is developing. To understand the difference between exercise as most of us saw it before and physical activity as how we should see it today, consider this quote from Robert Ornstein and David Sobel, authors of *Healthy Pleasures*: "Exercise is [a] usually deliberate, sometimes odious, sweat-soaked endeavor that can take time away from life, whereas physical activity can be any daily undertaking, work or play, that involves movement." Use this definition to monitor how physically active you are and to increase your level of activity as much as possible.

WALKING: THE BEST FORM OF REGULAR PHYSICAL ACTIVITY

The best way to begin boosting physical activity so that you stamp insulin resistance out of your life is simply to walk everywhere you can. Although walking may be frowned on by fitness fanatics, don't be discouraged: Walking is, evolutionarily speaking, the main type of exercise we were designed to do, and it is the best all-around form of physical activity for everyday living today.

The Advantages of Walking

Unlike some other forms of exercise, walking is always accessible: It does not cost anything to walk, and it can be done anywhere, without any special equipment other than a decent pair of shoes. Also, because walking is easy and convenient to do, people are much more likely to walk regularly than to stick with any other type of regular exercise program.

Walking also can be performed at low-, moderate-, and high-intensity levels, depending on which level suits you best. You can start out with a leisurely stroll, and you can continue increasing your stride and pace until you have a truly aerobic activity, or you can continue increasing your distance so that you have an exercise of endurance.

Finally, there is very little chance of becoming injured while walking. Walking is, in fact, the most injury-free exercise of all. No other type of physical activity has all of these advantages.

Creative Ways of Walking More

To incorporate more walking into your life, look for creative ways to put one foot in front of the other—both in everyday living and at special times, such as during vacations. Don't get into the rut of thinking you need to set aside a huge block of time to take one long walk. You can take several short walks throughout the day and get virtually the same health benefits.

Here, then, are some suggestions to step up the amount of walking in your life and to keep walking interesting. Some of these suggestions may seem like common sense, but many of us have automatically disregarded these as unimportant, when the truth is that every little bit of walking you do helps. You, of course, don't have to follow all of these suggestions. Just pick the ones you like best, and get started.

- Begin your day with a quick walk around the block, or make some time for a stroll during your lunch break. A quick walk does wonders for dealing with work stress: People experience decreased fatigue and tension for as long as 2 hours after taking a brisk 10-minute walk.
- Park your car at a spot farther away from work or the shopping center than you usually do, and walk the extra distance.
- At work, refrain from e-mailing coworkers, and walk down the hall or down a floor to deliver messages instead. (Don't laugh at this suggestion: It's been calculated that spending two minutes an hour to send e-mail to coworkers instead of walking down the hall to speak to them, day after day, could result in the gain of 11 pounds of fat over a decade!)
- Walk up stairs instead of taking the elevator, particularly if the floor you need to reach is the third floor or lower. If you haven't done this much, begin by walking down stairs, and eventually work up to walking up a flight or two.
- After work, walk at least to your mailbox, and better yet, walk around the block to relax and walk away any troubles you experienced at work.
- Ask a friend to join you for a walk, and then talk to him or her as you walk. When you are involved in good conversation, you often lose all track of time and distance.
- Ask your friend to go on a short hike with you, take a picnic lunch, and commune with nature. Again, you will probably have so much fun that you'll lose all track of how far you walk.

■ Combine a little romance with physical activity by going on regular moonlight walks with your significant other.

■ Take your baby for a stroll, and point out birds, flowers, animals, and other signs of nature along the way.

■ Take your kids to the zoo. You'll get a lot of walking in that way without even noticing it.

■ Walk your dog as often as you can; your dog will love you for it!

■ If a grocery store, convenience store, or drug store is within walking distance, save some gas, and get into the habit of walking to do your shopping and carrying your purchases home with you.

■ If the weather is bad outside, drive yourself to a shopping mall, and walk from end to end. If you look in the windows of stores as you pass by them, you can "preshop"—in other words, you can get an idea of what's available in different stores and then take note of which stores you'd like to go back to so you can take a closer look.

■ If you become bored with the places you regularly walk, take the time to drive yourself somewhere else—a park, a wilderness area, the beach, a downtown cultural area, or an amusement park. Soak in the sights and sounds of these new places, and enjoy yourself.

■ When vacationing, go to towns that have sightseeing areas or interesting places you can visit on foot. Walking through a new place you've never seen before is the best way to experience it firsthand.

OTHER FORMS OF PHYSICAL ACTIVITY FOR VARIETY AND FUN

Walking may be the best form of regular exercise, but it is certainly not the only way to get yourself moving just a little bit more. Any type of activity will do. What follows are more ideas on how to be more physically active—some ideas you may have thought about, others you might not have.

Recreational Bicycling

A leisurely ride on a bicycle is a great way to see a little more of the area around you. You can cover more territory on a bike than you can when you walk, and you can catch a lot of interesting sights and sounds. Most people experience the feeling of gliding through the air quickly on a bike as exhilarating and fun.

Don't feel as though you have to be a professional cyclist on the road to get benefits. Simply get on a bike and go at the pace that makes you feel most comfortable. Pedal for a while, then glide; pedal for a while, then glide. Make the ride interesting and enjoyable, so you'll want to ride the bike again.

In vacation spots, look for opportunities to rent bicycles, so you can see more of the area you're visiting. Something particularly fun to do on vacations is to rent a bicycle built for two and go pedaling with your spouse. You can talk about interesting things you see together along the way, and forget all about the exercise you're getting.

Dancing

Dancing to music that moves you is far more than physical activity: it is food for the body, mind, and soul. It exercises the whole body, and it can give as thorough an aerobic workout as any other strenuous exercise touted by fitness enthusiasts. It is never tedious and boring—it is just plain fun. Time has a way of flying when you're dancing.

When you are with a partner you adore, dancing can turn into a form of physical expression that goes beyond words. You can flirt with your partner, be playful or romantic, and show love to your partner—all at the same time you're exercising. What type of physical activity could be any better?

If you do not like to dance free-form to rock and roll, try taking classes of more structured dance, such as country swing, line dancing, folk and ethnic dancing, square dancing, or ballroom dancing such as the tango. Taking classes is a good investment because dancing moves are social skills you can use throughout your lifetime.

Better than choosing one type of dance to do is to learn several different types and vary the type you do, depending on your mood. When you do that, dancing will never become boring because there are almost limitless types of dancing to choose from.

Dancing is such a great social activity that some of us forget that dancing can be done solo, as well. This is great to remember if you don't have a partner, if you're self-conscious about dancing in public, or if the weather is bad and you just want to do some quick exercise in the privacy of your own home. Simply put on music that gets your toes tapping and move to the beat in whatever way feels best to you. Swing your hips, sway, hop—it does not really matter, just so long as you move. Don't feel as though you have to dance for 30 minutes straight. A dance here and a dance there definitely promotes health.

Swimming

Swimming is a great activity to add variety to your life, especially on a hot summer day. There's a feeling of freedom that comes from being buoyant and gliding through the water. Many people also experience a relaxing and often trancelike state from breathing in a rhythmic pattern.

Swimming often does not feel like exercise because the water cushions against stresses and does not leave you sweaty. Swimming gives the body a balanced workout because it exercises muscles of the upper body, as well as the lower.

Swimming is one of the best activities for anyone who has musculoskeletal problems, such as muscle injuries or arthritis. Exercising in water neutralizes the force of gravity, allowing free movement of muscles and joints.

Most of the time, it's easier to swim when you are on the road than when you're at home, unless you own a swimming pool or live in a condominium or apartment complex that has one. Most business-class hotels—as well as many motels—now have at least one swimming pool.

If you haven't plunged into this activity for a while, start slowly, moving through the water however it feels best. The backstroke, freestyle, and breaststroke are good choices for most people. Remember, though, that you are exercising muscles in your back and arms that you probably have not exercised much in a while, so go easy at first and don't overdo it.

Gardening and Lawn Work

Gardening is one of those activities that works your arms and back more than your legs, but there is a feeling of delight and centeredness that comes from working with the earth, planting seeds, and seeing your labor literally come to fruition.

Gardening serves a double purpose against Syndrome X if you grow nonstarchy vegetables such as lettuce, tomatoes, and cucumbers and fresh herbs in your garden. You should emphasize these foods, of course, in the Anti-X diet, and when you pull these foods straight out of the garden, they are at their peak of freshness, flavor, and healthfulness.

Interestingly, gardening comes close to approximating the type of activity our distant ancestors did foraging for food. Some of the best things about it, though, are the rewards you get for your efforts. Gardening provides you either with flowers that add beauty and color to your yard and life, or with fresh produce that you do not have to pay for and that tastes better than commercial produce—not a bad deal, while you're getting Anti-X physical activity in the process.

Few people enjoy lawn work—such as mowing the lawn or trimming hedges and trees—as well as gardening, probably because most people tend to think of lawn work as work more than play. It is a good form of exercise, though. Mowing the lawn, for example, combines walking and pushing for an all-over body workout. Consider using a manual mower—newer designs have made them lighter and easier to use, and they don't make a lot of noise and pollute like gas-powered mowers.

Probably the best thing about both gardening and lawn work is that they are done outside in the sunshine. Spending 15 minutes or so in the sunlight stimulates the body's production of vitamin D, a vitamin with strong Anti-X properties. (For more information on vitamin D, see Chapter 14.) Thus, doing moderate physical activity outdoors helps give you double protection against Syndrome X.

Other Ideas for Fun Activity

To become more active in still other ways, think about things you like to do that are fun and that give you pleasure. Remember your childhood, when you never even considered moving as "exercise"—it was "play" then. Remember that you can still play now, even though you're an adult.

A number of innovative physical activity programs focusing on "play" have been developed. One program, called Recess, is being offered by health clubs in New York City and Miami Beach. The object of the program is to once again do the fun and sometimes silly things we did as kids—activities such as twirling hula hoops, jumping rope, and running-backward races. You can do a Recess-type program at home: Just think about some activity you really loved doing as a kid, and re-create it.

Playing with your children is another creative way to move. Teach your child hopscotch, go fly a kite, or play catch with your child. You can also go horseback riding or sailing for a special outing. Your child will love you for this high-quality time together, and your body—as well as your mind and soul—will reap plenty of benefits, as well.

Other types of activities also make great play for adults. Dancing is one good social activity, but others that shouldn't be forgotten include bowling with friends and playing a game of golf in the great outdoors. (Golf, by the way, is a great opportunity to walk the course, rather than to drive in a cart.)

Look beyond obvious sports, though. *Charades*—a lively game in which a word or phrase that is to be guessed by others is acted out in pantomime—can really get your muscles moving and your heart pumping. It is a fun activity to try after a dinner with friends. Other ways to express yourself in pleasurable and physically active ways include "aerobic talking" (moving your hands when talking), giving your spouse a massage, or engaging in spirited lovemaking.

Vacations often offer opportunities to try fun activities that you typically can't do at home. Some examples include snorkeling in the Caribbean, taking hula lessons in Hawaii, or rowing a boat or canoeing on a mountain lake. Although you cannot do these activities all the time, experiencing them while on vacation adds to the fun and escape of getting away from your usual routine.

The bottom line with physical activity, of course, is to incorporate activity into daily living and to keep it fun and interesting. Cleaning the house and washing floors, for example, are activities virtually all of us do, but which most of us don't find to be fun. We can make them quite a bit of fun, though, if we change the routine by turning on the radio and scrubbing to the beat of the music, swinging our hips as we mop, or taking little time-outs away from cleaning for dancing breaks. The key is how you approach physical activity, and when you approach it creatively, time flies (and insulin resistance is held at bay) while you're having fun.

Putting This Chapter into Practice

Physical activity forces the body to burn more glucose and to use insulin more efficiently. Many of us don't have the desire to pursue structured exercises, such as jogging, aerobics, or body building, but being as physically active as possible is important.

- To help prevent insulin resistance and Syndrome X, engage in regular but fun activities, such as walking with a friend, swimming, dancing, and gardening.

- To reverse more entrenched symptoms of insulin resistance and Syndrome X, work up to a routine that includes some sort of daily physical activity. Keep it fun—go for longer walks, more laps in a pool, and longer nights of dancing.

PART THREE

The Anti-X
Supplement Plan

CHAPTER 11

Alpha Lipoic Acid:
The Master Nutrient

ALTHOUGH THE NAME *alpha lipoic acid* may sound a bit strange and unfamiliar, this vitamin-like nutrient is found in many foods, including spinach, broccoli, and beef. In fact, alpha lipoic acid (sometimes referred to as *lipoic acid* or *thioctic acid*) is so essential for health that small amounts of it are also produced by the body.

Of all the supplements that influence Syndrome X, alpha lipoic acid may be the single most important one. Its principal role is to help burn glucose, converting this sugar to energy that powers your heart, brain, and every other organ. Without sufficient alpha lipoic acid, your body could not muster any energy at all. Alpha lipoic acid has other functions, as well. It serves as one of the most distinctive antioxidant supplements, protecting the body against free-radical damage and also breathing new life into other antioxidants that have been used up fighting free radicals.

Researchers have known about alpha lipoic acid for many years, but only recently have they gained a good understanding of its diverse health benefits. Alpha lipoic acid was first isolated in the laboratory in 1951, and within a few years, German physicians began prescribing it for the treatment of *Amanita* mushroom poisoning and nerve disorders. In the early 1990s, taking a cue from American and European researchers, the German government approved alpha lipoic acid for the treatment of diabetic polyneuropathy, a very serious nerve disorder. We believe, however, that alpha lipoic acid's true potential lies in helping prevent and reverse Syndrome X and other glucose-related disorders.

FROM GLUCOSE TO ENERGY

Within each of the body's 60 trillion cells are thousands of micro-scopic *organelles*—microscopic organs—called mitochondria. These *mitochondria* are the powerful energy-producing factories of our bodies. They take in glucose and fats, process them, and gener-ate energy in the form of a chemical called adenosine triphos-phate (ATP). Mitochondria power each individual cell, and the collective energy of mitochondria in trillions of cells powers the entire body.

Most of this mitochondrial activity occurs during what biolo-gists call the "Krebs cycle," named after the scientist (Hans Krebs) who first described this process many years ago. You can picture the Krebs cycle as being somewhat like a wheel on a racing bike. As it spins around faster, it burns (or oxidizes) more glucose for energy. Many nutrients are involved in this process, including vita-mins B_1, B_2, and B_3. Alpha lipoic acid plays a key role in several places in the Krebs cycle, and studies have found that it (with other nutrients) spins the wheel more efficiently, increasing cellular energy levels.

Although alpha lipoic acid has been used to treat diabetic com-plications for many years, doctors did not understand exactly how it worked. In the 1990s, they identified a major reason why it bene-fits diabetics: *Alpha lipoic acid lowers glucose and insulin levels, reduces insulin resistance, and improves insulin sensitivity.* If alpha lipoic acid can help normalize glucose and insulin in full-blown diabetes, it can do the same in people with milder prediabetic conditions. Alpha lipoic acid's role in converting glucose to energy is crucial to its role in correcting insulin resistance and Syndrome X.

CONTROL YOUR GLUCOSE AND INSULIN

Although many physicians and researchers have raved about the multifaceted properties of alpha lipoic acid, we believe its most important role is in safely lowering glucose and insulin levels and improving insulin sensitivity (function). Back in 1970, researchers at the University of Pennsylvania noticed how alpha lipoic acid increased the burning of glucose. Since then, many animal exper-iments and well-controlled human studies have confirmed the glucose-controlling benefits of alpha lipoic acid. By increasing the burning of glucose and maintaining a normal insulin response, alpha lipoic acid corrects insulin resistance, the cornerstone of Syndrome X. The more glucose that is burned, the less insulin your body will have to secrete, and the less fat your body will be tempted to store.

Animal experiments by Erik J. Henriksen of the University of Arizona, Tucson, have confirmed that alpha lipoic acid infusions can increase the burning of glucose by one third. Other researchers, such as Nava Bashan of Ben-Gurion University of the Negev, Israel, have reported that alpha lipoic acid greatly stimulates cell uptake (and burning) of glucose, with the end result being a dramatic reduction in blood glucose levels. According to Bashan's animal experiments, alpha lipoic acid improved glucose uptake to the point that it was "comparable" to that of nondiabetic animals. In one series of experiments, glucose levels in diabetic rats decreased by a dramatic 23–45 percent.

Alpha lipoic acid increases the efficiency of insulin, which moves glucose into cells; it transports glucose into cells in ways independent of insulin; and it speeds up the Krebs cycle, so glucose is burned much more efficiently. Without the action of alpha lipoic acid, glucose remains in the blood, where it generates large numbers of dangerous free radicals and age-accelerating advanced glycation end-products (AGEs).

Human studies have found similar benefits from alpha lipoic acid. Supplements of 300 mg, taken twice daily, can lower glucose levels and improve the body's efficiency in burning glucose. High doses of alpha lipoic acid have also been found to improve insulin sensitivity—that is, insulin's effectiveness—by an average of 27 percent in overweight diabetic patients. This dramatic improvement is equivalent to a 27 percent reduction in insulin resistance—which would make a major impact on Syndrome X.

Stephan Jacob, a German physician and researcher, has conducted a number of small, scientifically controlled studies with diabetic patients. He has found that alpha lipoic acid (in dosages ranging from 600 mg to 1,800 mg daily) improved insulin sensitivity by about 30 percent. In addition, his patients gained greater glucose tolerance, meaning that they were better able to withstand the effects of dietary carbohydrates and sugars (although it is far better to concurrently reduce consumption of such foods). Another study by Jacob found that a single 1,000 mg dose of alpha lipoic acid temporarily increased insulin sensitivity by 50 percent!

IMPROVING GLUCOSE CONTROL

Alpha lipoic acid helps prevent Syndrome X in several ways:

- By reducing insulin resistance, the cornerstone of Syndrome X and diabetes
- By improving insulin sensitivity, so insulin functions more efficiently
- By lowering glucose levels (based on animal studies)
- By reducing the formation of AGEs
- By neutralizing free radicals

In addition to controlling glucose and insulin levels, alpha lipoic acid also limits the formation of AGEs, created when glucose damages proteins. High levels of AGEs accelerate the aging process, which increases susceptibility to most degenerative diseases. Sushil K. Jain, of the Louisiana State University Medical Center, Shreveport, has demonstrated how alpha lipoic acid raises levels of glucose-burning enzymes and doubles cells' ability to burn glucose. In addition, Jain found that alpha lipoic acid reduces levels of glycosylated hemoglobin, a standard marker of protein glycosylation (sugar-damaged proteins that age cells).

Alpha lipoic acid accomplishes all this not as a drug, but as a natural substance with normal roles in burning glucose for energy. The body's ability to produce alpha lipoic acid declines with age, so the body burns glucose less and less efficiently (which is partly why glucose levels tend to increase as people get older). In addition, eating a diet high in refined carbohydrates places a greater burden on the body's ability to burn glucose. Supplements restore more optimal levels of alpha lipoic acid, enabling glucose burning to proceed with more youthful efficiency. The effect, again, is to counteract Syndrome X.

None of this, however, means that alpha lipoic acid is a license to eat refined carbohydrates with abandon, or that it can "cure" diabetes. As part of a broader program that reduces the intake of refined carbohydrates, alpha lipoic acid can significantly lower glucose and insulin levels and improve insulin sensitivity.

ALPHA LIPOIC ACID: THE AMAZING ANTIOXIDANT

Glucose is a potent generator of free radicals, which cause much of the cell damage and complications associated with diabetes and Syndrome X. Alpha lipoic acid exerts its protective antioxidant

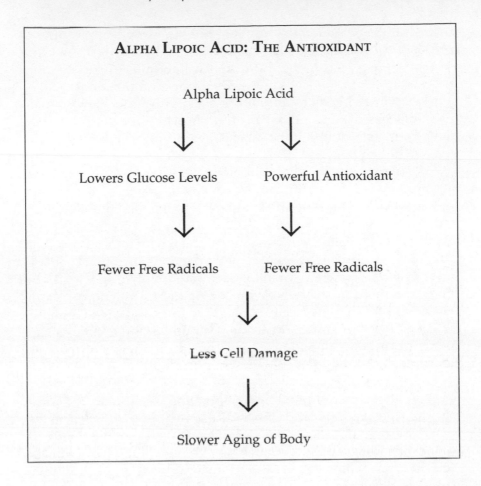

effects—that is, its ability to contain dangerous free radicals—in several distinctive ways. By lowering glucose levels in the blood-stream and improving insulin sensitivity, alpha lipoic acid greatly reduces a major source of free radicals.

There is also some evidence that alpha lipoic acid stems the production of free radicals in another fundamental way. Many free radicals are produced as a by-product of energy-generating free-radical reactions during the Krebs cycle in mitochondria. Although most of these free radicals are contained within the chemical reactions, a small number do leak out. Year after year, their damage accumulates. Alpha lipoic acid appears to tighten up these energy-generating chemical reactions and increase the containment of free radicals.

Alpha lipoic acid also functions as two different but related anti-oxidants—in effect, it's the Gemini of antioxidants. The best-known form, found in foods and supplements, is, simply, alpha lipoic acid. Lester Packer, a leading cell biologist at the University of California, Berkeley, has pointed out that it neutralizes hydroxyl free radicals, as well as singlet-oxygen radicals. Some alpha lipoic acid is converted by the body to another form, dihydrolipoic acid, which quenches peroxyl and peroxynitrite radicals. All of these are very dangerous types of free radicals, capable of inflicting considerable damage on the body.

As antioxidants go, alpha lipoic acid is almost unique in yet another respect. It can function in both the watery and the fatty regions of cells. This is significant because cells contain both watery and fatty media, and free radicals do damage in both areas. Nearly all other antioxidants work in one place but not the other. For example, vitamin E is fat-soluble and functions in the fatty membranes of cells, whereas vitamin C is water-soluble and works in the watery portions of cells. With the ability to function in both watery and fatty parts of cells, alpha lipoic acid can quench many different types of free radicals all over the cellular map, so to speak. In this way, alpha lipoic acid can quench many of the free radicals generated by glucose, mitochondria, and various metabolic processes.

As if all this were not enough, alpha lipoic acid plays a central role in what Packer calls the "antioxidant network." For many years, researchers believed antioxidants worked independently of each other, with vitamin E quenching certain types of free radicals, vitamin C quenching others, and so forth. It turns out that antioxidants are highly synergistic and work together.

A number of studies have found that groups of antioxidants have greater free-radical-quenching abilities than one would think from simply adding up the effect of individual antioxidants. Packer and his associates have confirmed that alpha lipoic acid plays a central role in the antioxidant network, helping to directly or indirectly recycle vitamins E and C, coenzyme Q_{10} (a vitamin-like substance), and glutathione (an antioxidant made by the body).

What's so important about recycling other antioxidants? Antioxidants get used up when they quench free radicals. Basically, their life is pretty much finished. By helping to recycle antioxidants, alpha lipoic acid breathes new life into them, lengthening their metabolic life span. Thus, antioxidants are interdependent and work best as a team. By strengthening the antioxidant network, alpha lipoic acid helps other antioxidants quench even more free radicals. (You'll read more about some of these antioxidants in the coming chapters.)

WHY ALPHA LIPOIC ACID IS A UNIQUE ANTIOXIDANT

- It quenches many different types of free radicals.
- It's more versatile than other antioxidants, working in both watery and fatty parts of cells.
- It strengthens the antioxidant network, bolstering vitamin C, vitamin E, coenzyme Q_{10}, and glutathione.

ALPHA LIPOIC ACID FOR NERVE DAMAGE

High glucose levels generate large numbers of free radicals, which damage cells, accelerate the aging process, and lead to the early onset of many diseases. One of the complications of diabetes is *neuropathy,* or damage to nerve cells, and it can take different forms. In some diabetics, it leads to considerable pain. In others, neuropathy causes numbness that prevents people from realizing that they are injured. Sixty percent of diabetics suffer some degree of nerve damage, from mild to severe.

For years, German physicians have used alpha lipoic acid to reverse diabetic nerve damage. More recently, researchers have found that alpha lipoic acid may benefit other types of nerve disorders. One such disorder is *sciatica* (pain in the sciatic nerve that runs down the leg), which is far more common (especially in the general population) than diabetic neuropathy. Because this type of nerve damage does not occur overnight, various types of "*preneuropathies*" probably coexist with prediabetic conditions, such as Syndrome X. The research indicates that alpha lipoic acid may forestall various types of nerve disorders in both diabetics and nondiabetics.

Alpha lipoic acid protects against nerve damage in several ways. One way is by restoring normal glucose levels. Conventional medical therapy often tries to accomplish this through intensive insulin injections, but the drawback is that these injections increase the risk of cardiovascular diseases. Alpha lipoic acid may be able to achieve the same result—without the side effects of insulin therapy.

Like all other cells, nerve cells are subject to free-radical damage. As an antioxidant, alpha lipoic acid can reduce this damage. One 1990s study found that alpha lipoic acid increased blood circulation, thereby facilitating delivery of more nutrients (and antioxidants) to nerve cells. Other research has found that alpha lipoic acid increases *nerve conduction*—that is, the speed of transmitted nerve signals. In diabetes and related glucose disorders, the speed of nerve signals slows down, interfering with normal nerve function. In a sense, alpha lipoic acid boosts the wattage of nerve cells and helps them communicate normally.

Abnormal nerve function can also affect the heart rate, leading to heart disorders. Studies in Europe and later at the Mayo Clinic in Minnesota have found that alpha lipoic acid can stabilize variable and erratic heart rates in diabetic patients. Physicians at the Mayo Clinic are also investigating—with promising preliminary results—how alpha lipoic acid can reverse nerve damage caused by toxic metal poisoning.

HOW ALPHA LIPOIC ACID CORRECTS NERVE DISORDERS

- It reduces free-radical damage to nerves.
- It improves the speed of nerve communication, thereby improving nerve function.
- It normalizes nerve sensitivity, reducing numbness or pain.

Sciatica is a fairly common condition among both diabetics and nondiabetics. In a 1990s animal study, British researchers compared alpha lipoic acid with high-tech recombinant human nerve growth factor (rhNGF) in the treatment of sciatic nerve pain. Both alpha lipoic acid and rhNGF raised levels of some desirable neurotrophic compounds, which aid nerve-cell communication. However, only alpha lipoic acid boosted levels of a key neurotrophic substance, called neuropeptide Y-like immunoreactivity, in the sciatic nerve. Increasing this neurotrophic substance should improve nerve function and reduce sciatic pain.

It is important to recognize that other nutrients also work with alpha lipoic acid in maintaining normal nerve function. Many animal and human studies have found that gamma-linolenic acid (GLA), a fatty acid the body makes from dietary oils, can also protect against diabetic neuropathy. Contemporary studies have found that a combination of alpha lipoic acid and GLA work even better than alpha lipoic acid alone.

In one experiment, Norman E. Cameron, of the University of Aberdeen, Scotland, gave diabetic rats GLA, alpha lipoic acid, or both nutrients. While GLA and alpha lipoic acid each led to some improvements in nerve function, the combination had a "marked synergistic action," increasing both nerve-signal speed and blood flow.

Although people should make their own GLA from linoleic acid (found in vegetable oils and nuts), they don't always. Diabetics (as well as people who have eaten a lot of processed and packaged food that contains partially hydrogenated oils) have trouble converting linoleic acid to GLA. Supplements of evening primrose or borage oil provide preformed GLA and are helpful in such cases.

THE ANTIAGING EFFECTS OF ALPHA LIPOIC ACID

Alpha lipoic acid can reverse a great many other signs of age-related physical and mental deterioration. Once again, it works by reducing glucose and glucose-generated free radicals, protecting cells from free radicals generated by other sources, and increasing cellular energy levels. Without sufficient energy, cells lose the oomph they need to perform at their best.

Cataracts

A number of intriguing animal studies have found alpha lipoic acid to reduce the risk of *cataracts,* which are characterized by areas of permanent cloudiness in eye lenses. Cataracts are strongly associated with both elevated glucose and overexposure to sunlight. Both glucose and sunlight generate free radicals, which damage lens proteins and form AGEs.

One of the key antioxidants in the fluid surrounding the eye is glutathione. Alpha lipoic acid is very good at boosting the body's production of glutathione. Alpha lipoic acid contains sulfur, a very important dietary mineral, which is a building block of glutathione.

In one experiment, alpha lipoic acid prevented the development of cataracts in 60 percent of the animals exposed to a chemical known to damage the lens. In a German study, researchers found that alpha lipoic acid prevented the formation of cataracts in rats, even when they were exposed to a high-calorie (diabetes-causing) diet. The cataracts were blocked in part because alpha lipoic acid increased the levels of glutathione in the eye.

Stroke

Lester Packer believes that one of the most important uses for alpha lipoic acid may be to minimize damage due to strokes. Stroke is a major cardiovascular disease and a leading cause of death and disability. Typically, a clot in a blood vessel in the brain interrupts blood flow, suffocating brain cells. When blood flow resumes, huge numbers of free radicals are formed, which inflict still more damage to brain cells. In one experiment by Packer, stroke deaths among laboratory rats dropped from 78 percent to just 26 percent after administration of alpha lipoic acid.

THE HEALTH BENEFITS OF ALPHA LIPOIC ACID

- As a powerful antioxidant, it quenches age-accelerating free radicals.
- As a glucose and insulin regulator, it benefits people with Syndrome X and diabetes.
- By increasing the burning of glucose, it increases energy levels.
- By quenching free radicals, it can reduce the risk of cataracts.
- As an enhancer of liver function, it can detoxify poisonous mushrooms and other toxins.

ALPHA LIPOIC ACID AND ITS EFFECTS ON OTHER DISORDERS

Alpha lipoic acid has many other significant health benefits that, while unrelated to its roles in maintaining normal glucose and insulin function, are noteworthy. One of its most remarkable—and, unfortunately, overlooked—uses is in the treatment of *Amanita* and *Galerina* mushroom poisoning. Among the pioneers in using alpha lipoic acid in the treatment of mushroom poisoning are Fred Bartter, chief of Hypertension and Endocrinology at the National Institutes of Health, and Burt Berkson.

Each year, hundreds of people become gravely ill after picking and eating wild mushrooms that look safe and edible. Toxins in these mushrooms inhibit normal liver function and destroy liver cells. In general, the prognosis for people who eat a lethal dose of poisonous mushrooms is not very good. Most people endure tremendous pain, slip into a coma, and die. The most desirable conventional treatment is a liver transplant. There are not enough livers for all the people who need one, however, and liver-transplant surgery is always risky and expensive.

Alpha lipoic acid does not seem to directly neutralize mushroom toxins. Instead, it bolsters and maintains liver function in the face of very destructive toxins. As alpha lipoic acid does this, abnormally high levels of liver enzymes (such as SGPT) return to normal. Not surprisingly, alpha lipoic acid can help patients manage chronic hepatitis infections, as well.

This liver-protective action of alpha lipoic acid is significant because the liver is the body's chemical processing and detoxification factory. When people are exposed to toxic chemicals, such as carbon monoxide, paint fumes, formaldehyde fumes from new carpeting, and even alcohol, their livers become stressed, and there is an increased potential for abnormal glucose metabolism. Alpha lipoic acid supplements help the liver defend itself and do its job to detoxify these chemicals and help regulate glucose levels.

HOW TO FIND AND USE ALPHA LIPOIC ACID

For years, researchers believed that the richest dietary sources of alpha lipoic acid were those body organs in which mitochondria are densely abundant. At the top of the list were beef and some organ meats (e.g., heart). Although these are excellent sources of alpha lipoic acid, recent experiments by Lester Packer have found that spinach may be the richest food source of this nutrient. Broccoli also contains large amounts of alpha lipoic acid.

Although Popeye may have had the right food in mind for increasing his strength, the bioavailability of alpha lipoic acid from food may not be that straightforward, according to Packer. The potential problem, he has explained, is that alpha lipoic acid in food is bound to a protein called lipoyllysine. Protein-bound alpha lipoic acid may not be as biologically active as the "free" form found in supplements.

The convenience and safety of alpha lipoic acid supplements enables people to "load" this important nutrient to optimal levels. For healthy people, 50–100 mg daily should be sufficient. This dose of alpha lipoic acid is available in tablet and capsule form at nearly all health-food stores and vitamin shops. Alpha lipoic acid is also added to many antioxidant formulas that contain vitamins E and C and other nutrients.

To help correct glucose intolerance and Syndrome X, 100–300 mg daily may be needed. These higher doses can improve glucose metabolism and insulin sensitivity. Hypoglycemic (low blood sugar) reactions are rare because alpha lipoic acid acts to lower and stabilize glucose and insulin levels. Although blood tests can document the effect of alpha lipoic acid, subjective feelings of greater well-being may be the best judge.

Diabetics can benefit from 300–600 mg of alpha lipoic acid, with the higher dose being best for people who suffer complications such as neuropathy. However, diabetics taking insulin or hypoglycemic drugs should take high doses of alpha lipoic acid under a physician's guidance because alpha lipoic acid supplements may reduce their drug requirements.

Putting This Chapter into Practice

- To help prevent Syndrome X, take 50 mg of alpha lipoic acid daily, preferably as part of a multivitamin or antioxidant supplement (that also contains vitamins E and C and other antioxidants).

- To reverse problems relating to glucose intolerance and Syndrome X, dosages ranging from 100 to 300 mg of alpha lipoic acid daily may be beneficial. Diabetics are likely to benefit from 600 mg daily, but they should take this high dose under the guidance of a physician. High doses of alpha lipoic acid may reduce requirements for medications that lower glucose levels.

CHAPTER 12

Vitamin E:
The Cardiovascular
Nutrient

LIKE ALPHA LIPOIC ACID, vitamin E also influences glucose and insulin levels. However, it plays a much more significant role as an antioxidant that counteracts many of the unwanted health effects of free radicals, including those generated by excess glucose.

Discovered in 1922, vitamin E is the body's principal fat-soluble antioxidant. That means it quenches free radicals in the body's fatty structures, such as cell membranes and cholesterol. By stemming the formation of free radicals, vitamin E reduces the age-accelerating, disease-promoting effects of diabetes and Syndrome X. Most dramatically, this nutrient can prevent coronary heart disease, one of the key diseases caused by Syndrome X.

VITAMIN E, GLUCOSE, AND INSULIN

Diabetics—and people with Syndrome X—commonly suffer from *oxidative stress* (the general condition defined by abnormally high levels of free radicals), which plays havoc with the body's management of glucose levels. Vitamin E supplements can reduce oxidative stress—and improve glucose control.

Vitamin E helps manage glucose and insulin in several ways. First, it helps shield cells from the toxic effects of glucose. Glucose increases free-radical damage to cells, alters normal cell replication, and literally kills cells. Vitamin E strengthens cells and helps them resist these assaults.

Second, vitamin E offsets some of the effects of elevated insulin. High levels of insulin deplete vitamin E levels in the body. The reason is not entirely clear, but it is possible that elevated levels of the hormone speed up chemical reactions that promote free-radical formation and drain vitamin E reserves. The consequence should be obvious: People with Syndrome X or diabetes will have a higher than normal requirement for vitamin E.

If this greater need for vitamin E is not satisfied, people are more likely to suffer higher levels of free-radical damage, which in turn will accelerate the development of cardiovascular disease, Alzheimer's disease, cancer, and other degenerative diseases. Vitamin E can help protect against these diseases.

Third, taking vitamin E supplements can reduce glucose levels and restore more normal insulin function. In 1999, Giovanni Davi, of the University of Chieti School of Medicine, Italy, reported that daily doses of 600 IU (international units) of vitamin E reduced glucose levels and free-radical formation in diabetic patients in just two weeks. His patients also benefited from significant reductions in thromboxane B_2, a compound that promotes blood clots and increases the risk of heart disease. Similarly, Giuseppe Paolisso, of the University of Naples, Italy, found that vitamin E supplements improved glucose tolerance and insulin function in healthy people, as well as in diabetics.

Animal studies have echoed these findings. In an experiment with overweight rats, supplemental vitamin E reduced glucose and free-radical levels to those typical of lean rats. In another study, vitamin E improved insulin sensitivity—that is, it reduced insulin resistance—in rats fed large amounts of fructose.

Vitamin E has other benefits related to improved glucose control. By quenching free radicals, it reduces the formation of glycosylated proteins, which speed the aging process and the progression of degenerative diseases. One type of glycosylated protein, glycosylated hemoglobin in the bloodstream, is the standard measure of diabetic control. High levels of glycosylated hemoglobin indicate that glucose levels are out of control. Vitamin E supplements can help diabetics do a better job of managing their glucose, and they can probably help protect healthy people from Syndrome X.

HOW VITAMIN E HELPS IN SUGAR-RELATED DISORDERS

- It protects cells from many of the harmful effects of glucose.
- It reduces glucose levels.
- It improves insulin sensitivity.
- It neutralizes free radicals.
- It prevents glycosylation of proteins.

STAYING YOUNGER WITH VITAMIN E

Both glucose and insulin accelerate the aging process and, with that, the risk of all age-related diseases. Vitamin E slows the aging process, largely by preventing free-radical damage to genetic material (such as deoxyribonucleic acid, or DNA) and cell membranes. It also puts the brakes on the aging process by limiting the formation of glycosylated proteins and AGEs, which damage normal proteins and healthy cells.

Marguerite M. B. Kay, of the University of Arizona School of Medicine, Tucson, has investigated how vitamin E affected "band 3" proteins, which are essential for transporting nutrients into cells. Band 3 proteins cease functioning when they are damaged by free radicals. In experiments with laboratory mice, Kay confirmed that the breakdown of band 3 proteins led to the aging of brain and immune cells. Then she gave mice the equivalent of 400 IU of vitamin E daily. The vitamin E delayed the deterioration of these important proteins.

In another study, Katalin G. Losonczy, of the National Institute of Aging, analyzed the vitamin-supplement-taking habits of 11,000 elderly people. People who were long-term users of vitamin E supplements were 60 percent less likely to die of coronary heart disease and 59 percent less likely to die of cancer, compared with people who did not take the vitamin. Decreasing the risk of heart disease and cancer translates into a longer, healthier life.

WHY VITAMIN E IS GOOD FOR THE HEART

Glucose intolerance, Syndrome X, and diabetes greatly increase the risk of heart disease. With the prevalence of sugar-related disorders, it is no surprise that heart disease is the leading cause of death in the United States and other Western nations.

Vitamin E's greatest health benefit is its ability to turn back the clock on your heart and blood vessels—in effect, making them younger and more resistant to disease and the deleterious effects of excess glucose and insulin. It protects the cardiovascular system in many different ways.

▪ As a fat-soluble antioxidant, vitamin E works where fats and free radicals can cause problems. It prevents free-radical oxidative damage to the low-density lipoprotein (LDL) form of cholesterol. This is significant because LDL is one of the more dangerous subtypes of cholesterol, and oxidized LDL is strongly associated with Syndrome X. By preventing LDL oxidation, vitamin E neutralizes a key risk factor for heart disease.

▪ Vitamin E blocks some of the early steps in the formation of cholesterol deposits in blood vessel walls. According to research by Ishwarlal "Kenny" Jialal, of the University of Texas Southwestern Medical Center, Dallas, vitamin E inhibits an inflammatory process that starts to damage blood-vessel walls. It also prevents cholesterol deposits from forming in those walls.

▪ Vitamin E turns off the gene that programs the growth of smooth-muscle cells in blood-vessel walls. (Free radicals turn on this gene.) Smooth-muscle cells, along with cholesterol, form part of the lesion that narrows the opening of blood vessel walls, leading to reduced blood flow and heart disease.

▪ Vitamin E is also a mild *anticoagulant,* meaning that it prevents abnormal blood clots, which can cause heart attacks and strokes. It reduces the activity of several compounds that promote blood clots, including thromboxane. However, vitamin E does not usually amplify the effect of prescription anticoagulant drugs, such as warfarin.

▪ Vitamin E normalizes the ability of blood vessels to dilate— that is, to widen in diameter and relax. This periodic relaxation is essential for the normal give and take needed to help pump blood. When blood vessels cannot relax, the risk of cardiovascular diseases increases.

▪ Vitamin E prevents free-radical oxidation to internal and external cell membranes, or walls. These membranes are rich in polyunsaturated fatty acids (PUFAs), making them especially susceptible to oxidation. When membranes become damaged, they prevent nutrients from moving into cells and waste products from moving out of them, thereby disrupting normal cell function. Oxidized cell membranes are characteristic of older cells, and they are more likely to malfunction than are younger membranes.

■ Vitamin E reduces free-radical damage to DNA, the molecule that forms your genes and chromosomes. Less genetic damage means that heart (and other) cells can replicate more accurately, and more accurate replication means the body can produce younger-acting, disease-resistant cells for more years.

VITAMIN E REDUCES THE RISK OF HEART DISEASE

It may surprise you to learn that Canadian physicians first described vitamin E's benefits to the heart in the 1940s. Spurred by clinical successes with several patients, Evan Shute and his colleagues in London, Ontario, began prescribing vitamin E to more patients with cardiovascular diseases. They briefly described their results in a letter published in the scientific journal *Nature,* and the June 10, 1946, issue of *TIME* magazine heralded Shute's finding as a cure for heart disease. Although Shute and his cardiologist brother Wilfrid treated tens of thousands of patients with vitamin E over the next 30 years, their work was largely dismissed by conventional physicians.

Why was the Shutes' discovery ignored by medicine? Under the best of circumstances, medicine is a very conservative profession and is usually slow to accept new ideas. When Evan Shute first described the heart benefits of vitamin E, most physicians simply could not imagine how or why vitamin E would benefit the heart. Shute had the misfortune of recognizing the heart benefits of vitamin E a decade before scientists had figured out that antioxidants influenced human health, and more than two decades before vitamin E was recognized as an essential nutrient for people.

In 1993, two studies, published simultaneously in the *New England Journal of Medicine,* started to change opinions about vitamin E. Meir J. Stampfer and Eric B. Rimm reported that nurses taking at least 100 IU of supplemental vitamin E had a 41 percent lower risk of heart attack, compared with women not taking supplements. Similarly, male physicians taking at least 100 IU of vitamin E daily were 37 percent less likely to suffer a heart attack.

Other researchers were encouraged by these findings. Howard N. Hodis, of the University of Southern California School of Medicine, Los Angeles, tracked the progress of patients who had undergone bypass surgery and were taking a prescription drug to reduce their risk of further heart disease. He found that patients who took

100–450 IU of vitamin E—of their own accord—developed smaller cholesterol deposits, compared with patients not taking supplements. Because Hodis had carefully documented the size of cholesterol deposits, it was a clear demonstration that vitamin E could slow the development of coronary heart disease—one of the primary consequences of Syndrome X.

The most persuasive vitamin E study so far, published in the British medical journal *Lancet,* exceeded nearly all expectations for vitamin E. Nigel G. Stephens and his colleagues at Cambridge University gave either placebos or 400–800 IU of natural vitamin E daily to 2,000 patients with documented heart disease. (Later in this chapter, we discuss the difference between natural and synthetic vitamin E.) The results were astounding. The incidence of nonfatal heart attacks dropped by 77 percent in the vitamin E group!

Several 1990s studies have found that vitamin E supplements can even circumvent serious dietary abuses. Gary D. Plotnick, of the University of Maryland School of Medicine, Baltimore, looked at how a McDonald's breakfast, high in fats and refined carbohydrates, interfered with the ability of blood vessels to dilate. Blood vessels need to periodically relax in order to properly move blood through the circulatory system. When they fail to relax (a condition sometimes described as *endothelial dysfunction*), blood cannot flow normally, and the risk of heart disease increases. Endothelial dysfunction is common in Syndrome X.

Plotnick fed 20 healthy men and women a breakfast consisting of a McDonald's Egg McMuffin, Sausage McMuffin, and two hash-brown potato patties. The high-fat meal raised the subjects' level of triglycerides—one of the characteristic symptoms of Syndrome X—by more than 60 percent and substantially decreased normal endothelial function for up to four hours. In other words, a single breakfast greatly increased the risk of a heart attack for hours! When the subjects were also given supplements of vitamins E (800 IU) and C (1,000 mg), they were protected against these changes.

The lesson in all this? Most people are eating diets high in both refined carbohydrates and fats. These diets lead to a range of abnormalities, from elevated glucose and insulin levels to abnormal blood-vessel behavior. Vitamin E blocks many of these effects. While we don't want to encourage anyone to eat a bad diet and simply pop vitamins, vitamins E and C offer people considerable protection against dietary lapses.

> ## *FIVE WAYS VITAMIN E PROTECTS AGAINST HEART DISEASE*
> - It quenches dangerous free radicals.
> - It prevents free-radical damage to cholesterol.
> - It prevents the formation of cholesterol deposits.
> - It prevents the growth of artery-clogging smooth-muscle cells.
> - It reduces the risk of blood clots.

VITAMIN E AND ALZHEIMER'S DISEASE

Virtually every degenerative disease is caused, or exacerbated, by free radicals, many of which spin off elevated levels of glucose or from the incomplete burning of glucose. A number of studies have found vitamin E to protect against free-radical damage to brain and nerve cells and to fight neurological disorders.

In the most dramatic study conducted along these lines to date, Mary Sano, of the Columbia University College of Physicians and Surgeons, New York, investigated whether vitamin E or the drug selegiline slowed the final slide into end-stage Alzheimer's disease. Sano and her colleagues gave 341 Alzheimer's patients 2,000 IU of vitamin E (a very high dose!), selegiline, both the vitamin and the drug, or a placebo daily for two years.

Vitamin E worked the best, delaying the onset of end-stage Alzheimer's disease by almost eight months, compared with patients taking the placebo. Although vitamin E did not improve the patients' thinking processes, it did enable them to continue performing basic activities (such as eating, grooming, and using a toilet) longer than other patients.

Sano and other Alzheimer's researchers believe that vitamin E works by curbing free-radical damage to brain cells. Alzheimer's is characterized by a tangle of amyloid protein around brain cells, which essentially chokes them to death. Free radicals promote the proliferation of amyloid protein, and by curbing this action of free radicals, vitamin E loosens this protein's grip on brain cells.

The American Psychiatric Association has gone on record recommending vitamin E as a key treatment for Alzheimer's disease. We go a step further: We believe that vitamin E is so important in maintaining normal brain function that people should start taking it when they are still young, to delay the earliest stages of free-radical damage to brain cells. Also, by taking it well before the first signs of

Alzheimer's appear, a lower and less costly dose (such as 400 IU daily) should be sufficient.

> ### MAJOR DISEASES VITAMIN E BENEFITS
> Diabetes and other glucose disorders
> Coronary heart disease
> Alzheimer's disease
> Immune deficiencies
> Cancer

VITAMIN E, IMMUNITY, AND CANCER

High levels of glucose reduce the ability of immune cells to fight infections. Not surprisingly, diabetics—people with the highest glucose levels—are more prone to infections than are nondiabetics. Because the development of most diseases is a gradual process, prediabetic conditions, such as Syndrome X, probably increase the risk of infection.

A faltering immune system may also lose its ability to identify and destroy cancer cells. High levels of glucose and insulin are associated with an increased risk of at least some cancers, such as those of the biliary tract, lung, colon, liver, pancreas, breast, and endometrium.

Immune function typically decreases with age, just as glucose levels tend to increase, and this may be part of the reason why people become more susceptible to infections and cancers as they get older. A healthy immune system protects against infectious microorganisms and cancers, and vitamin E enhances these defenses.

Vitamin E and Infections

The immune-enhancing effect of vitamin E has been clearly demonstrated by Simin Nikbin Meydani, of Tufts University. Meydani gave 88 elderly men either a placebo or 60 IU, 200 IU, or 800 IU of vitamin E daily for four months. She then measured the men's immune function with a skin test called the "delayed-type hypersensitivity skin response." The test measures how quickly or slowly the immune system responds to a challenge from a vaccine or an *antigen* (a substance that stimulates an immune response). The faster the response, the better the immune system.

While vitamin E did not improve the immune response against every type of challenge, it still had an impressive effect. The men averaged a sixfold increase in antibodies in response to hepatitis B and tetanus antigens. The most impressive effect of vitamin E, however, may have been that noted in a passing observation by Meydani. The three groups of men taking vitamin E reported having 30 percent fewer infections, compared with men taking the placebo.

An animal experiment, also by Meydani, may explain why vitamin E reduced infections. Vitamin E increased the numbers of "natural killer" cells, a powerful type of immune cell, and lowered the concentrations of flu viruses in laboratory mice. While vitamin E may not be a cure for the common cold or flu, it can definitely bolster resistance to infection.

Vitamin E and Cancer Prevention

Free-radical damage to DNA is also one of the chief underlying causes of cancer. This link may explain why high levels of glucose are associated with an increased risk of some types of cancer.

Dozens of population-based studies have noted that people who consume large amounts of antioxidants (usually through fruits and vegetables) have a lower risk of cancer, compared with people who consume small amounts of antioxidants. Antioxidant supplements can also reduce the risk of cancer. In the 1990s, researchers at the Fred Hutchinson Cancer Research Center, Seattle, analyzed 59 studies on vitamin and mineral supplements and cancer risk. Overall, the researchers concluded, supplements did reduce the risk of several types of cancer. Vitamin E turned out to be the supplement most consistently related to a lower risk of cancer.

This benefit of vitamin E has been borne out in both human and animal studies. For example, men who take vitamin E supplements are one third less likely to develop prostate cancer, compared with other men. Similarly, there is compelling evidence from animal studies showing that vitamin E supplements can lower the risk of breast cancer.

LITTLE KNOWN BUT HELPFUL TYPES OF VITAMIN E

Before you begin taking vitamin E, it's helpful to know a little more about this amazing nutrient. There are actually eight different types of vitamin E molecules. The most common type found in nature is alpha-tocopherol. It is also the type most efficiently absorbed by people because the body's binding and transport proteins prefer it over all other forms.

However, the other tocopherols also possess antioxidant properties, and they probably have worthwhile, though minor, roles in health. For example, gamma-tocopherol is more effective than alpha-tocopherol in quenching some types of free radicals.

Alpha-, beta-, delta-, and gamma-tocotrienols are also considered minor parts of the vitamin E family of molecules. Research has found that the tocotrienols do have health benefits relevant to Syndrome X and diabetes. Tocotrienol supplements (200 mg daily) can reduce cholesterol levels. In one study, subjects benefited from declines of 15 percent in cholesterol, 8 percent in LDL cholesterol, 25 percent in thromboxane, and 12 percent in glucose.

THE DIFFERENT TYPES OF VITAMIN E

Tocopherols	Tocotrienols
Alpha-tocopherol	Alpha-tocotrienol
Beta-tocopherol	Beta-tocotrienol
Delta-tocopherol	Delta-tocotrienol
Gamma-tocopherol	Gamma-tocotrienol

EXERCISE INCREASES VITAMIN E NEEDS

Regular physical activity improves virtually all symptoms related to Syndrome X and diabetes. It also increases the burning of glucose and fat, as well as the formation of muscle, which further improves glucose and fat burning. However, there is a danger in overexercising. Studies by Lester Packer, of the University of California, Berkeley, and other researchers have found that strenuous exercise can increase production of unwanted free radicals. So while exercise is extremely beneficial, steps have to be taken to minimize its few negative effects.

Günter Speit and his colleagues at the University of Ulm, Germany, documented that overexercising generated enough free radicals to damage DNA in the white blood cells of five volunteer subjects. However, when the men took 1,200 IU of vitamin E daily before undergoing a rigorous treadmill test, all DNA damage was prevented. The lesson is clear: Exercise, but also take your vitamin E.

HOW TO BUY AND USE VITAMIN E

Vitamin E is the one supplement that everyone, sick or well, should be taking. Because of extensive food refining and processing, the modern diet is practically devoid of vitamin E. At the same time, diets high in sugars and other refined carbohydrates and in processed vegetable oils generate huge numbers of destructive free radicals and increase vitamin E requirements.

Buying the best kind of vitamin E supplement, however, can sometimes be a little tricky, so it is important to understand what's available at health-food stores and pharmacies.

Natural versus Synthetic Vitamin E

Vitamin E is available in natural and synthetic forms. Although companies selling the synthetic form claim there is no difference between the two, there *is* a significant difference. Natural vitamin E has a different chemical structure from the synthetic version, and it is far superior. The human body selects for natural vitamin E over synthetic.

How do you tell the difference? Just look at the fine print on the back of the label. Natural vitamin E is identified by its chemical name, which will be some variation of "d-alpha-tocopherol." The key thing to look for is the "d," which indicates the natural vitamin E molecule. In contrast, synthetic vitamin E is identified with a "dl."

LOOK FOR THE NATURAL "d" IN VITAMIN E

Natural vitamin E has twice the potency of the synthetic vitamin. To tell the difference, read the fine print on vitamin bottles. Natural vitamin E will be identified as "d-alpha-," as in d-alpha-tocopherol, d-alpha-tocopheryl acetate, or d-alpha-tocopheryl succinate. Think of the natural "d" as "desirable."

Synthetic vitamin E is identified with "dl-alpha-," as in dl-alpha-tocopheryl acetate. Think of the synthetic "dl" as "don't like."

Milligram for milligram, or pound for pound, natural vitamin E is far better absorbed than the synthetic form, and it seems to do a better job in the body. Apparently, the body's means of assimilating and transporting vitamin E prefers the structure of the natural molecule.

The body prefers natural vitamin E by a wide margin. For years, researchers believed that natural vitamin E was 1.36 times more potent than synthetic vitamin E. To equalize the two types of vitamin E, a common standard was developed. As a result, all vitamin E is measured in international units, or IU.

The differences between natural and synthetic vitamin E go beyond this distinction, however. The original studies describing the 1.36 difference between natural and synthetic vitamin E were based on animal studies. Recently, U.S. and Canadian researchers conducted experiments to determine which form of vitamin E was best absorbed by humans.

Their findings left few doubts. They discovered that a range of people, men and women, healthy and sick, absorbed *twice* as much natural vitamin E as the synthetic. Their bodies also retained natural vitamin E longer than the synthetic. Looked at another way, synthetic vitamin E is absorbed only half as well as natural vitamin E. The difference is so great that 400 IU of natural vitamin E is far more potent than 400 IU of synthetic vitamin E.

At the health-food store or pharmacy, synthetic vitamin E may cost less than the natural, and it may be tempting to save a couple of dollars, but this is truly one of those situations where you get exactly what you pay for. Our advice: When shopping for supplements, look for the "d" indicating natural vitamin E.

Different Types of Natural Vitamin E

Once you find natural vitamin E at the store, you'll discover there are several types. Although each is an excellent product, one may be better than others in preventing or treating certain conditions. The following information may seem a little technical, but it is important to know the pros and cons of different types of vitamin E to select the one best for you.

■ *D-alpha-tocopherol* is one form of natural vitamin E that is well absorbed, but a little less stable over the long term than other natural vitamin E products. However, long-term stability should not be a problem with d-alpha-tocopherol if you store it in a cool, dry place and use it up within a year or so.

■ *D-alpha-tocopheryl acetate* is another natural form of vitamin E. The acetate in the name comes from the fact that this type of vitamin E has been combined with a molecule related to vinegar to improve its shelf life and stability. D-alpha-tocopheryl acetate definitely has a proven track record: It is the form of the vitamin most often used to prevent and to treat heart disease.

■ *D-alpha-tocopheryl succinate* is another natural form of vitamin E. It is very stable and has a long shelf life, and it has also been used to reduce the risk of heart disease. Based on animal studies, d-alpha-tocopheryl succinate also seems to have some distinctive anticancer properties.

■ *"Mixed natural tocopherols"* form the supplement that most resembles what's actually found in nature. When produced the right way, this type of product contains a specific amount of d-alpha-tocopherol, along with modest amounts of natural beta-, gamma-, and delta-tocopherols.

■ *Tocotrienols*, discussed earlier, can have a role in reducing cholesterol levels. However, tocotrienols do not behave in the same way as tocopherols, so they should be taken only in addition to natural vitamin E, not as a replacement for it.

For the vast majority of people, 400 IU daily of natural vitamin E should be sufficient. Lower amounts are less effective in reducing the risk of heart disease. Higher amounts, such as 800 IU daily, do a better job of preventing free-radical damage to cholesterol, but a combination of different antioxidants (including alpha lipoic acid, vitamin C, and beta-carotene) may accomplish this and provide broader health benefits. Because vitamin E is fat soluble, it should be taken with a little food.

Putting This Chapter into Practice

■ To help protect against Syndrome X, diabetes, and heart disease, take 400 IU of natural ("d-alpha") vitamin E daily.

■ To help reverse these conditions, take 400–800 IU of natural vitamin E.

CHAPTER 13

Vitamin C:
The Well-being
Nutrient

Vitamin C, also known as ascorbic acid, plays diverse roles in health and disease prevention. It protects against Syndrome X, diabetes, and their accompanying disorders in many different ways. It works most directly by blocking many of the deleterious effects of elevated glucose and insulin.

In addition, as a powerful antioxidant, vitamin C quenches free radicals generated by glucose and other sources, such as immune cells. In doing so, it reduces the free-radical damage that contributes to heart disease, cancer, and other age-related degenerative diseases. One sign of severe vitamin C deficiency is a tendency toward bruising—common in diabetes—caused by collagen-weak blood-vessel walls leaking blood into surrounding tissues.

THE GLUCOSE–VITAMIN C CONNECTION

Glucose and vitamin C possess nearly identical chemical structures (glucose: $C_6H_{12}O_6$ versus vitamin C: $C_6H_6O_8$). For most animals, this similarity has been a godsend. For humans, the situation has resulted in biochemical confusion and has increased the risk of diseases caused by excessive glucose.

Nearly all mammals convert glucose to vitamin C in the liver or kidneys, providing a ready supply of this essential substance. Indeed, most animals produce prodigious amounts of vitamin C, the equivalent of 2,000–13,000 mg daily in an adult human. Under stress, animals increase their production of vitamin C still further. These higher levels of vitamin C help maintain *homeostasis*—that is, they keep an animal's body on an even keel. In other words, glucose serves a very important purpose besides being a source of energy.

The story is different for people. Millions of years ago, a genetic mutation occurred in an early primate, preventing it from making its own vitamin C. Somehow this creature survived, probably because it had access to abundant dietary vitamin C. It reproduced, and its descendants evolved, with all of them inheriting this defect. For these descending species—which include human beings—vitamin C became a dietary nutrient essential for survival.

The consequence of this evolutionary accident helped lay the genetic foundation for glucose intolerance, Syndrome X, and diabetes: People are capable of having high levels of glucose in the bloodstream without any biological purpose for it. The buildup of glucose starts to resemble unwanted gang members hanging around on a street corner and up to no good. Too much glucose, which might otherwise be converted to vitamin C, overstimulates insulin production and generates large numbers of dangerous free radicals.

Competition between Glucose and Vitamin C

Given the similar chemical structures between glucose and vitamin C, it is not surprising that these two molecules compete against each other. To continue the analogy, they become like rival gangs fighting over the same cellular turf. Indeed, there is considerable evidence that insulin aids the transport of vitamin C into cells, just as it assists glucose. Both want to ride on the insulin transport molecule, and competition between glucose and vitamin C is inevitable.

The implications of this competition are serious. When the bloodstream is flooded with glucose (because of the consumption of refined carbohydrates), vitamin C has difficulty gaining a foothold. Furthermore, when cells become insulin resistant, it is conceivable that they also become vitamin C resistant. If this is the case, insulin resistance would interfere with how cells use both glucose *and* vitamin C.

Not surprisingly, diabetics are frequently deficient in vitamin C, even when they get modest amounts through their diets. Study after study has shown that low vitamin C levels are intertwined with and contribute to diabetic complications, including heart disease, kidney disease, and eye disorders. Syndrome X is the prediabetic condition in which vitamin C levels have already been compromised.

Replenishing vitamin C through supplementation seems to edge out some of the glucose (though it is best, as we have recommended, to also reduce the glucose load by avoiding dietary sugars and other refined carbohydrates). One study found that 2 grams (2,000 mg) daily of vitamin C lowered both glucose and glycosylated hemoglobin levels. Vitamin C also normalizes insulin function. Researchers at Arizona State University, Tempe, have reported that the same dose of supplemental vitamin C delayed the insulin response to glucose. The result is a more normal, less trigger-happy insulin response to glucose.

Vitamin C benefits diabetics in other ways. Many diabetic complications result from the body's overproduction of *sorbitol,* another sugar. Sorbitol levels go up in diabetics, increasing levels of *aldose reductase,* an enzyme that has a hand in many diabetic complications. Vitamin C supplements reduce both sorbitol and aldose reductase, and the vitamin appears to be at least as good as pharmaceutical aldose reductase–inhibiting drugs. Again, bear in mind that diabetes does not develop overnight, and that glucose intolerance and Syndrome X precede it.

HOW VITAMIN C IMPROVES GLUCOSE TOLERANCE

- It lowers glucose.
- It normalizes insulin's response to glucose.
- It neutralizes free radicals.
- It reduces glycosylated hemoglobin.

Vitamin C also slows the aging process that high glucose and insulin accelerate. It does this in a couple of ways. Vitamin C is the body's principal water-soluble dietary antioxidant, and it quenches the hydroxyl free radical, considered the most dangerous of all radicals. Vitamin C also reduces the glycosylation of proteins, including AGEs, which, as the acronym suggests, age cells.

As one illustration, free radicals and AGEs promote the formation of *cataracts,* a common eye disorder in the elderly, which diabetics are more prone to developing. One recent study found that women taking supplements of 400 mg or more of vitamin C for 10 years were 80 percent less likely to develop cataracts.

VITAMIN C PROTECTS AGAINST INFECTION

Diabetics are more susceptible to infection than are nondiabetics, and people with prediabetic conditions, such as Syndrome X, probably also suffer impairments in immunity. Relatively modest increases in glucose levels interfere with the function of white blood cells and antibodies, which are programmed immune-system responses to specific types of infection.

Vitamin C helps the immune system in several ways. White blood cells and T cells need large amounts of vitamin C to function. During an infection, immune cells have to work extra hard, and their vitamin C reserves are quickly depleted. When immune cells lose their vitamin C, they become less effective in fighting bacteria and viruses. Vitamin C supplements help optimize the function of immune cells. In addition, vitamin C may help tissues resist bacterial and viral attackers by strengthening the body's skin and tissues, reinforcing a physical barrier.

Vitamin C also protects the body's cells against an immune backlash. White blood cells destroy bacteria in what biologists call the "free-radical burst." After engulfing bacteria, white blood cells literally detonate free radicals to destroy the bacteria. (That's another example of the lethal nature of free radicals.) Unfortunately, free radicals often leak out (sort of like peripheral blast damage) and injure nearby cells. The situation is exacerbated when vitamin C levels are low because inadequate antioxidant reserves limit the body's ability to clean up these excess free radicals. Supplemental vitamin C helps the body clean up these unwanted free radicals.

Like alpha lipoic acid and vitamin E, vitamin C enhances the body's total antioxidant network. This network consists of vitamin E, alpha lipoic acid, glutathione, and other antioxidants. Together, these antioxidants form a powerful team that can bolster the body's ability to deal with stresses, such as infections.

VITAMIN C'S BENEFICIAL EFFECTS ON IMMUNITY

- Vitamin C boosts the activity of immune cells, so they do a better job of fighting bacteria and viruses.
- Vitamin C helps the body maintain homeostasis so infections are fewer and less severe.
- Vitamin C helps clean up excess free radicals, which the immune system uses to fight germs.

VITAMIN C AND HEART DISEASE

Cardiovascular diseases are the leading cause of death in North America, and heart disease is a primary consequence of Syndrome X. Perhaps surprisingly, as much as 40 percent of a person's risk of cardiovascular disease may be related to his or her overall intake of different antioxidants, according to Joel A. Simon, of the Veterans Affairs Medical Center, San Francisco. Vitamin C plays a critical role in maintaining the health of the heart and cardiovascular system. In a study of more than 6,600 men and women, Simon and his colleagues found that the people with the highest blood levels of vitamin C were 27 percent less likely to suffer from heart disease and 26 percent less likely to have a stroke.

Vitamin C influences the heart in many different ways. As you recall, one of the characteristics of Syndrome X is an abnormal cholesterol profile. Total cholesterol levels become elevated. In addition, levels of the good high-density lipoprotein (HDL) form of cholesterol decrease. This decrease in HDL alters the ratio between the bad low-density lipoprotein (LDL) form of cholesterol and HDL—in effect, raising LDL levels. Furthermore, free-radical oxidation of LDL increases. Each of these changes increases the risk of coronary heart disease.

Studies dating back to the 1970s have demonstrated that supplemental vitamin C can reduce overall cholesterol levels. More recently, researchers have reported that supplements improve a person's overall cholesterol profile, shifting it from one that is characteristic of Syndrome X to one more resistant to coronary heart disease. For example, researchers at the University of Sydney, Australia, have shown that taking 1,000 mg of vitamin C for four weeks can decrease LDL cholesterol by 16 percent. (If LDL was 150 mg/dl, the drop would be a significant 24 mg/dl.) Other studies have demonstrated that vitamin C can prevent the free-radical oxidation of LDL, reducing another risk factor for heart disease. At the same time, high blood levels of vitamin C are associated with increases in desirable HDL cholesterol.

Vitamin C also prevents the microcirculatory (circulation in the smallest blood vessels) changes induced by cholesterol. This is important because many cardiovascular diseases originate in the smallest blood vessels of the body. (For example, the heart contains its own network of smaller blood vessels.) In an experiment with rabbits, Swedish researchers found that a high-cholesterol diet reduced blood flow and increased blood clotting in the smallest blood vessels (arterioles and conjunctival vessels). When vitamin C was added to the diet, blood flow was almost the same as in rabbits fed a normal (non-cholesterol-containing) diet.

Hypertension, also part of Syndrome X, might also be eased with ample vitamin C intake. Although studies do not show a direct cause-and-effect relationship, they do show a strong association between high blood levels of vitamin C and normal blood pressure.

VITAMIN C'S BENEFICIAL EFFECTS ON THE HEART

- Decreases total cholesterol
- Lowers the bad LDL cholesterol
- Raises the good HDL cholesterol
- Enables blood vessels to relax
- Lowers blood pressure
- Controls free-radical activity and damage
- Reduces the risk of blood clots

Elevated cholesterol levels interfere with the normal *vasodilation*, or relaxation, of blood vessels. Healthy blood vessels periodically relax in order to move blood through the circulatory system. When they don't relax (endothelial dysfunction), the stage is set for high blood pressure and coronary heart disease. Vitamin C, however, promotes blood-vessel relaxation in both diabetics and nondiabetics. Furthermore, just as high-fat meals cause endothelial dysfunction, supplemental vitamin C (1,000 mg) and vitamin E (800 IU) protect against it.

Vitamin C may protect the heart in yet another way. When vitamin C levels are low, the collagen that holds together blood-vessel walls is more likely to become damaged under the force of normal blood pressure (and more so if blood pressure is high). Vitamin C reinforces the structure of blood-vessel walls.

VITAMIN C, DNA DAMAGE, AND CANCER

All cancers arise from uncorrected damage to DNA, the molecules that form genes and chromosomes. DNA contains the biological instructions that tell the body's cells what to do, such as which enzymes or proteins to produce and when to divide and create a new cell.

Free radicals from glucose and other sources can damage DNA and introduce the equivalent of typographical errors in these instructions. Although DNA repair mechanisms identify and correct most errors, they are as fallible as any proofreader. Some of the errors are inevitably overlooked. These mistakes accumulate with time and are passed on to new cells, which suffer additional DNA damage. As the number of typographical errors increases, the original instructions become less and less clear. Sometimes, the instructions are rewritten in such a way that cancer cells arise and proliferate.

Many studies have demonstrated that antioxidants, including vitamin C, reduce the rate of DNA damage. In doing so, antioxidants slow the accumulation of age-related cell damage and reduce the risk of cancer. Studies in the 1990s have found that vitamin C reduces DNA damage and actually plays a key role in repairing DNA damage.

In clinical practice, large doses of vitamin C—10,000 mg or more daily—can have a powerful, beneficial effect on patients with cancer. Vitamin C sharpens the immune response to cancer, strengthens the collagen of healthy tissue in a way that bolsters its defense against invading cancer cells, and has a marked *analgesic* (pain-reducing) effect.

HOW VITAMIN C REDUCES THE RISK OF CANCER

- It prevents damage to DNA, so fewer abnormal cells are created.
- It enhances immune function, so the body can identify and destroy cancer cells.
- It strengthens collagen, so tissues are more resistant to invading cancers.

HOW TO BUY AND USE VITAMIN C

There's a lot of controversy surrounding how much vitamin C a person needs. The official recommended amount is a scant 60 mg daily, although some researchers have argued that the government-recommended amount should be increased to 200 mg daily. Both of these amounts fall far short of what we believe people should be getting.

Any way you slice the data, vitamin C deficiency is disturbingly common by RDA standards. A recent study of 500 patients receiving routine exams at medical clinics in the Phoenix area found 30 percent of them to have low levels of vitamin C in their blood and 6 percent to be seriously deficient in the vitamin. The normal blood levels were based on the consumption of 60 mg of vitamin C daily. If the norm had been set higher, such as 200 mg daily, many more of the patients would have been found deficient.

The principal dietary reason for these deficiencies is that people are not eating many fruits and vegetables, the foods richest in vitamin C. Public-health recommendations call for the consumption of at least three to five servings of fruits and vegetables daily to reduce the risk of heart disease and cancer, but most people fall far short of that. Different studies have found that only 9, 17, or 34 percent of people consume three to five servings of fruits and vegetables daily. Whichever number you happen to pick, the vast majority of North Americans do not eat many vitamin C–rich foods.

When you go a step further and take into consideration that our evolutionary requirements for vitamin C probably equal those of vitamin C–producing animals, the officially recommended amount of vitamin C is ridiculously low. It is simply impossible to get 2,000 to 13,000 grams of vitamin C from the diet. The only way to obtain these amounts of vitamin C, and to compensate for the genetic defect that prevents people from making their own vitamin C, is to take supplements.

Vitamin C supplementation enhances the body's defenses against excess glucose and glucose-derived free radicals. Based on the evidence, vitamin C also lowers cholesterol levels and blood pressure, thereby reversing some of the characteristics of Syndrome X.

There is a huge range of individual requirements, with the variation related to genetics, lifestyle habits, and stress. Your optimal dose of vitamin C is probably somewhere between 2,000 and 4,000 mg daily. You may require more vitamin C during the acute phase of an illness. For a short time, 10,000–20,000 mg daily is permissible. As you start to recover, you may decrease your dose to regular intake levels.

There are many different forms of vitamin C on the market, and choosing one over another really comes down to cost and personal preferences. Most supplemental vitamin C is ascorbic acid made from corn, though some is synthesized from other plants (such as beets). Some products also contain rose hips and bioflavonoids, and these are important nutrients. However, plain old ascorbic acid is usually the least expensive. Do read labels carefully for other ingredients, which may include sugar. In general, you will find health-food store brands to be free of sugars.

Many other nutrients play important roles in protecting people from Syndrome X. In the next chapter, we explore the beneficial roles of dietary minerals, such as chromium, zinc, and others.

Putting This Chapter into Practice

- To increase your resistance to Syndrome X, and for overall well-being, take 1,000–2,000 mg of vitamin C daily.
- To reverse Syndrome X, take 2,000–4,000 mg of vitamin C daily. Higher dosages may bolster immunity (which is compromised by glucose) and reduce symptoms of colds and other infections.

CHAPTER 14

Chromium, Zinc, Magnesium, and Other Minerals

LIKE ALPHA LIPOIC ACID, vitamin E, and vitamin C, many minerals perform important functions in the prevention and treatment of Syndrome X (and its accompanying health complications). Minerals occur in the simplest of chemical forms and are tiny in comparison to vitamins. Even though they're minute in size, however, they can play big roles in regulating glucose and insulin function.

Sixteen minerals are currently considered essential to health. Certain ones—such as chromium, zinc, and magnesium—stand out in their ability to help regulate glucose and help insulin to function more efficiently. This chapter explains the primary benefits of these key minerals and runs down the benefits—and drawbacks—of others.

CHROMIUM

Chromium is without a doubt the most important mineral for the prevention and treatment of insulin resistance and Syndrome X. It is so important for proper glucose and insulin function that chromium supplements are a must for virtually everyone in Western nations. Ninety percent of U.S. residents don't receive adequate amounts of chromium from their diets, and this pattern probably holds true for other North Americans and Europeans. Furthermore, many people eat excessive amounts of sugar and refined grains, which deplete chromium levels. It's little wonder that insulin resistance and Syndrome X are becoming more prevalent.

The symptoms of chromium deficiency are actually the symptoms of Syndrome X—elevated glucose, insulin, and cholesterol; elevated triglycerides; and decreased levels of the good HDL cholesterol. Because a lack of chromium can cause all these conditions, it shouldn't be surprising that supplemental chromium can help improve all these conditions. Chromium accomplishes all this by helping address the root of the problem—faulty insulin function.

Chromium and Insulin Function

Chromium's key benefit is that it helps insulin function more efficiently. This means that chromium is helpful for people with all types of glucose and insulin disorders—not just people with glucose intolerance and diabetes, but also people with *reactive hypoglycemia* (those who experience quick blood-sugar highs, followed by quick blood-sugar lows—a condition considered a precursor to diabetes). In people with hypoglycemia, supplemental chromium normalizes insulin function, leading to increased insulin efficiency and a return to normal glucose levels more quickly after a high sugar intake. In people with high glucose, improved insulin efficiency leads to more efficient removal of sugar from the blood. Chromium, therefore, can be considered a blood-sugar balancer, as well as regulator.

A person's response to chromium is related to his or her degree of glucose intolerance. While 200–400 mcg supplemental chromium is often all that is needed to improve the glucose levels of people with mild insulin resistance, higher dosages may be needed to elicit the greatest therapeutic effects for people with adult-onset diabetes.

To get an idea of how effective chromium supplementation is for people with insulin resistance, consider the results of a well-designed 1997 study. One hundred eighty people with adult-onset diabetes were given twice-daily doses of either a dummy pill, 100 mcg chromium picolinate, or 500 mcg chromium picolinate, and their blood glucose and insulin levels were monitored after two and four months. The group that took 200 mcg per day had their fasting and two-hour insulin levels decrease, but they experienced no improvement in blood-glucose levels. In contrast, the group taking 1,000 mcg per day experienced what can only be described as "spectacular" results—a drop in glucose and insulin levels to near normal after just four months! Medications could not have achieved these results—clear proof that supplemental chromium can help reverse insulin resistance and Syndrome X quickly, not only in people with moderate insulin resistance but also in people with severe insulin resistance.

Chromium, Fat Loss, and Body Composition

By helping to increase insulin sensitivity and to lower high insulin levels, chromium also aids fat loss and weight control. In a study of 154 subjects who were provided no advice on weight loss, diet, or exercise, those given daily chromium picolinate supplements for two months experienced a significantly greater reduction in body-fat percentage and indirect measurements of fat weight than those given a placebo. Without any other dietary alterations, the use of chromium picolinate supplements resulted in a loss of about 0.5 pounds of body fat per week! In another study, the use of supplemental chromium (400–600 mcg daily) together with supplemental L-carnitine (200 mg daily), an increase in fiber intake (by eating more fruits and vegetables), and a moderate restriction of calories resulted in even more impressive fat loss.

Chromium has other benefits for people trying to slim down and firm up. It can maintain lean muscle tissue when calorie intake is low. Even when a person doesn't restrict calories, chromium can increase a person's total lean body mass, which in turn increases metabolism and the body's ability to burn fat. It also can help reduce sugar cravings, which are common among people with Syndrome X. Through all these different mechanisms, chromium supplements help people lose fat and improve body composition, especially when used in conjunction with the diet and physical activity program outlined in this book.

Chromium, Blood Fats, and Blood Pressure

Chromium is important for fat metabolism (as well as carbohydrate metabolism), and a number of studies have found that chromium supplements have beneficial effects on blood fats, such as decreasing total cholesterol and LDL cholesterol, increasing beneficial HDL cholesterol, and decreasing triglycerides. A double-blind, placebo-controlled study found that dietary supplementation with chromium picolinate for two months lowered blood levels of triglycerides in diabetics by an average of 17.4 percent. Because elevated triglycerides and elevated cholesterol are risk factors for cardiovascular disease, chromium's ability to favorably influence these levels make the mineral important in the prevention of cardio-vascular disease, especially for diabetics, who are at increased risk.

Chromium's ability to augment insulin sensitivity also makes it helpful for the treatment of another component of Syndrome X— high blood pressure. Intake of sugar typically raises systolic blood pressure, but in experiments with spontaneously hypertensive rats, chromium picolinate supplements overcame the typical sugar-induced elevations in blood pressure—at least up to a point. The best strategy for correcting hypertension, of course, is to take chromium supplements *and* to reduce sugar intake.

The Antiaging Effects of Chromium

Chromium also slows the aging process. Animals deprived of chromium have shorter life spans, while animals supplemented with chromium picolinate live 37 percent longer than they would in their natural habitat.

To understand why chromium helps delay aging, remember that diabetes is a model of accelerated aging. The high glucose levels characteristic of diabetes generate large amounts of free radicals, and excess free radicals are involved in virtually all diseases of aging—from heart disease to cataracts. High glucose also greatly increases the risk of glycosylation—the damaging reaction in which sugar sticks onto proteins in our cells, damaging and destroying them.

Chromium, of course, increases insulin efficiency and very effectively lowers high glucose levels, ultimately decreasing the free radicals and AGEs that quite literally age us. By enabling insulin to transport glucose from the bloodstream into the cells more efficiently, chromium promotes youthful cell performance and helps prevent premature aging.

Supplementing with Chromium

The amount of supplemental chromium you should take depends on your state of health and glucose levels. For the general prevention of Syndrome X, 200 mcg of chromium picolinate daily should be sufficient. If you have any one of the conditions involved in Syndrome X—obesity, hypertension, unhealthy cholesterol or triglyceride profiles, or diabetes—or if these conditions run in your family, increase your supplemental intake to 400–800 mcg chromium picolinate daily. This amount also can be helpful if you have hypoglycemic symptoms, including strong cravings for sugar. For optimal absorption, split the dose up, so you take two or three smaller doses daily.

If you have Type 2 diabetes, take 1,000 mcg of chromium picolinate daily. This recommendation, though, comes with a caveat: If you are taking medication to control your glucose, start with 200 mcg chromium per day for a week, and monitor your glucose levels closely. Continue to increase the amount of chromium you take by 200 mcg per week until you reach 1,000 mcg, and then have your physician adjust your medication accordingly. Supplemental chromium works so well at improving insulin function that less medication to control glucose usually is needed. This is a good thing—it indicates a reversal or lessening of the insulin resistance you have—but it also means that you need to carefully monitor your glucose levels to avoid overmedicating yourself and experiencing an acute low-blood-sugar episode.

Chromium has been studied extensively and has been found to be extraordinarily safe in people, even when given in very high doses. However, a couple of small cell-culture studies have found that extremely high doses of chromium picolinate can cause chromosome breaks, which, according to a handful of researchers, may increase the risk of cancer. The dosages used in these studies were thousands of times higher than a person would take supplementally; indeed, virtually everything is dangerous at a high enough dose. We're confident the amounts of chromium picolinate we recommend are preventive and therapeutic, not harmful. If you would prefer to take a different type of chromium, such as chromium chelate, though, look over the selection and choose one in a health-food store.

ZINC

Zinc, the second most abundant trace mineral in the body, plays critical roles in glucose regulation, the proper function of insulin, and weight control. A number of present-day factors have caused zinc deficiencies to become quite common. These factors include modern agricultural and food-processing practices that have caused the zinc content in our food supply to plummet, and the recent trend for Americans to avoid zinc-rich meats in favor of low-zinc processed convenience foods and vegetarian foods.

Unfortunately, deficiencies of zinc put people at greater risk for Syndrome X. A recent study of 3,575 rural and urban adults found that the prevalence of coronary artery disease, diabetes, and glucose intolerance was significantly higher among those consuming lower intakes of dietary zinc. This same study also found that as zinc intakes rose among subjects, there was a significantly lower prevalence of hypertension, high triglyceride levels, low HDL levels, and abdominal obesity. These, of course, are all components of Syndrome X.

Zinc and Insulin Function

The link between zinc deficiency and Syndrome X makes sense when you consider zinc's role in insulin function. Zinc is needed to help the pancreas produce insulin, to allow insulin to work more effectively, and to protect insulin receptors on cells. In healthy individuals, you will recall, insulin is secreted from the pancreas after carbohydrates are eaten, and this hormone lowers glucose levels in the blood and drives sugar into the cells, where it can be used as fuel for energy.

When zinc levels are low, two things can happen. One, the pancreas may not secrete adequate amounts of insulin, so glucose levels remain high. Two, the insulin that is released may not work as effectively as it should. When this happens, glucose cannot enter cells and remains elevated in the blood. The body typically responds to high glucose levels by pumping out more and more insulin in an effort to lower glucose levels, but the insulin doesn't work properly, so insulin levels rise and stay high. When this happens, Syndrome X and the cascade of health problems that accompany it can result.

Zinc and Weight Control

Zinc deficiency also appears to be involved in the development and perpetuation of obesity, which can be both a symptom and a consequence of Syndrome X. As mentioned, inadequate levels of zinc can interfere with the normal cellular response to insulin; high insulin levels, in turn, promote fat storage in the body. When insulin levels are high, it's virtually impossible to keep weight off—or to lose weight—because of the powerful effect of insulin.

Zinc also may help weight control and help reverse Syndrome X because it is an *antagonist* of copper (i.e., it competes with copper for intestinal absorption and protein binding sites in the blood). This is significant because in test tube and animal experiments, excess copper increases fat (or triglyceride) synthesis from sugar. Zinc supplementation lowers copper levels, so it may decrease the synthesis of triglycerides, which can show up as either triglycerides in the blood or fat on the body.

Zinc, Appetite, and Body Composition

Zinc may also be involved in the development of obesity and Syndrome X because it affects blood levels of *leptin,* a hormone that influences appetite, energy expenditure, and possibly body composition. Supplementation of 30–60 mg of zinc added to people's daily diets increases their blood levels of leptin, while men who are fed zinc-deficient diets produce less leptin. Leptin is produced in fat cells, and it signals the state of energy stores to the brain, telling us when to eat and when to put down the fork. If leptin levels are low from an inadequate zinc intake, we may never feel full or may continue to have food cravings and overeat. Overeating nutrient-poor carbohydrates, of course, is one of the primary dietary contributors to the development of Syndrome X.

Zinc deficiency can contribute to overweight another way, too: Even marginal zinc deficiencies are associated with decreased *lean body mass* (the muscular part of the body, as opposed to the fat part). Zinc supplementation in people who are zinc deficient, on the other hand, has increased their lean body mass, while their fat mass has either remained stable or decreased. Researchers hypothesize that by raising leptin levels, zinc supplementation may help body composition, signaling the body to build lean tissue and either keep fat mass stable or possibly lower it.

Zinc levels in both the blood and the tissues of obese individuals are often markedly lower than those in people of normal weight. This means that maintaining good zinc reserves—or rebuilding zinc reserves if you're low—may be a critical and significantly overlooked factor for staying slim, or for losing weight and keeping it off—which are important factors in preventing the development of Syndrome X.

Supplementing with Zinc

Zinc is vital for normal glucose metabolism and insulin function, and most Americans don't consume even the Recommended Dietary Allowance (RDA) for zinc, which is probably too low for optimal glucose management and health. Zinc supplements, therefore, are a necessary addition to any nutritional regimen designed to prevent and reverse Syndrome X. Zinc picolinate, zinc aspartate, zinc chelate, zinc citrate, and zinc monomethionine all appear to be good forms of supplemental zinc. In contrast, zinc sulfate should be avoided because, in some people, it can be irritating to the stomach. Optimal amounts of zinc vary widely among individuals, but 30 mg daily is a good dose for most people.

The tricky part in taking zinc supplements is whether to take copper with zinc, as is typically recommended. Zinc and copper are antagonists, so too much zinc can cause a copper deficiency, which sometimes can cause undesirable changes in good HDL and bad LDL cholesterol ratios. For this reason, nutritionally oriented practitioners often advise taking copper along with zinc in a 10:1 to 15:1 ratio of zinc to copper. However, people who have Syndrome X have been found to have low zinc levels. When zinc levels are low in the body, copper remains unchecked and tends to build up, and high copper levels are a risk factor for cardiovascular disease.

Research also shows that diabetics have higher copper levels and lower zinc levels than people who don't have diabetes, and diabetics with complications such as retinopathy, hypertension, or microvascular disease have higher copper levels than diabetics without complications. As mentioned earlier, excess copper increases fat synthesis from sugar, so people with high glucose, hypertension, or obesity probably should steer clear of a lot of supplemental copper. (We explain more about copper shortly.)

MAGNESIUM

Magnesium is another mineral critical for the prevention and treatment of Syndrome X. At least half of all Americans do not consume the RDA for magnesium (320 mg for women; 420 mg for men), and low amounts of magnesium in the diet greatly increase the risk of developing Type 2 diabetes—which, of course, is insulin resistance at its worst.

Magnesium deficiency appears to be one of the factors that pave the way for the development of Type 2 diabetes. One study that followed about 14,000 middle-aged people for up to seven years found that men and women with the lowest levels of magnesium in their blood at the start of the study were twice as likely to be eventually diagnosed with diabetes, compared with those with the highest levels of magnesium.

Magnesium and Insulin Function

The link between magnesium deficiency and adult-onset diabetes isn't surprising: Magnesium plays several central roles in the normal function of insulin. It is necessary for the production and release of insulin; it is also required by cells for maintaining insulin sensitivity and increasing the number of insulin receptors. Without adequate magnesium levels within body cells, insulin becomes less effective at moving glucose from the blood into the cells, and diabetes can result.

Magnesium supplementation is an important aid for many people with glucose intolerance and insulin resistance. In one study of nonobese older subjects, magnesium supplements (400 mg elemental magnesium per day) improved insulin response and action, and glucose handling. This means that magnesium can help prevent and reverse insulin resistance and Syndrome X.

Magnesium and High Blood Pressure

Just as adequate levels of magnesium protect against the development of diabetes, they also appear to help prevent another common consequence of insulin resistance—high blood pressure (or hypertension). Population studies have found that when magnesium intake is high, blood pressure is lower. Magnesium supplements have also been found to be helpful in the treatment of many cases of hypertension.

Magnesium probably helps prevent and reverse high blood pressure in several ways. First, it helps insulin work more effectively, which in turn helps to prevent high insulin levels, a strong risk factor for high blood pressure. Second, the mineral helps relax blood vessels. Third, sufficient magnesium is needed for the cells of the body to maintain normal levels of potassium. People with high blood pressure—and insulin resistance in general—tend to have low levels of potassium and elevated levels of sodium within their cells. Magnesium activates the cellular membrane pump that pumps sodium out of, and potassium into, the cell; it probably lowers blood pressure in this way.

Magnesium and Protection against Syndrome X Complications

Magnesium helps prevent several devastating complications of insulin resistance, Syndrome X, and diabetes—including cardiovascular disease, the number-one killer of men and women in the Western world. Just as low magnesium intakes are linked to high blood pressure, they're also linked to higher rates of heart disease and stroke.

Magnesium is absolutely essential for the proper functioning of the heart and the entire cardiovascular system. It improves heart rate and reduces arrhythmias. It also keeps blood platelets from clumping together and forming blood clots, and this in turn helps protect against both heart attack and stroke. Bear in mind that if you have any symptom of Syndrome X, you're much more at risk for developing cardiovascular disease. Taking supplemental magnesium is one important step to help prevent its development.

Maintaining a high intake of magnesium also appears to be protective against another devastating complication of diabetes—*retinopathy*, damage to the blood vessels of the retina. Low levels of magnesium are correlated with the development and progression of this condition, which can lead to severe vision problems and blindness.

Supplementing with Magnesium

Because magnesium helps insulin efficiency, virtually everyone who has Syndrome X or is prone to it can benefit from magnesium supplementation. For most people, a good dose is 400 mg daily. Excellent forms of the mineral include magnesium oxide, magnesium chloride, magnesium carbonate, magnesium citrate, magnesium malate, magnesium aspartate, and magnesium lactate.

Vitamin B_6 works together with magnesium in many enzyme systems, and it increases the intracellular accumulation of magnesium. So, to increase magnesium in the cells (which is where you really need it), make sure to take a B-complex vitamin that contains at least 30 mg of vitamin B_6 in addition to supplemental magnesium.

Diabetics have higher needs for magnesium, and they also excrete more magnesium than do healthy people, so if you're diabetic, you may benefit from amounts up to 800 mg (400 mg twice daily). The only caution is if you have juvenile-onset diabetes, diabetic kidney disease, or other kidney dysfunction—these conditions can cause impaired excretion of mineral salts, so if you have any of these conditions, consult your physician before taking magnesium supplements.

OTHER MINERALS OF IMPORTANCE

Manganese

Manganese, a trace mineral, acts as a cofactor in various enzyme systems that help the body utilize vitamin C and some B vitamins and that facilitate glucose metabolism. In guinea pigs, a deficiency of manganese results in diabetes and the frequent birth of off-spring that develop abnormalities in the pancreatic secretion of insulin. Manganese supplementation completely reverses these abnormalities.

Little research has been conducted on manganese in humans, but it's been reported that oral manganese supplements significantly lowered blood glucose levels in one diabetes patient who was unresponsive to insulin. Nutritionally oriented practitioners, though, have been using supplemental manganese, along with chromium and zinc, to successfully treat insulin resistance and Type 2 diabetes for years.

To help prevent Syndrome X, consider taking 10 mg manganese daily. Diabetics have only half the manganese of normal individuals, so if you have documented high glucose levels or any other symptoms of Syndrome X, up to 30 mg per day may be needed.

Selenium

Selenium does not directly affect glucose or insulin function, but it is important for those with Syndrome X because it works synergistically with vitamin E and helps it do a better job. Selenium also is an important component of two key enzymes—glutathione peroxidase, which scavenges free radicals, and thioredoxin reductase, which recycles vitamin C. Selenium, in other words, strengthens the network of antioxidants that protect the body from the ravages of free radicals, and people who have high glucose levels generate excessive amounts of free radicals. Animal experiments have shown that supplemental selenium helps reduce the oxidative stress that is part and parcel of diabetes.

Selenium also helps boost immunity and appears to play a protective role against the development of heart disease and cancer. As we discussed in Chapter 3, people who have high glucose levels have weakened immune systems and are much more prone to heart disease and cancer. Therefore, supplemental selenium (100–200 mcg in the form of sodium selenite or selenomethionine), in conjunction with vitamin E, appears to be good assurance against free-radical buildup and the development of degenerative diseases. This applies to everyone, but especially to those with insulin resistance. Because high doses of selenium may be toxic, don't take more than 400 mcg daily—a very safe dose.

Vanadium

Vanadium is showing up in an increasing number of nutrient supplements, but there are pros and cons associated with its use. The mineral has been found to have impressive beneficial effects in diabetics: Animal studies have found that vanadium lowers fasting glucose in diabetic mice and also lowers LDL cholesterol, triglyceride levels, and blood pressure. Vanadium works by mimicking insulin, thereby helping cells to absorb sugar more effectively. In other words, vanadium can help overcome insulin resistance, which is the core of Syndrome X.

That's the good news. The bad news is that vanadium hasn't yet been demonstrated to be an essential mineral for humans, it may cause adverse health consequences such as depression and kidney problems in very large doses, and it seems to act more like a drug than a nutrient needed for health. All this means that vanadium should be used extremely cautiously.

Consumers should also know that some researchers believe that because vanadium mimics insulin, it may turn off pancreatic cells that make insulin. This suggests that if you take large amounts of supplemental vanadium for a long period of time, and then stop, your body may underproduce insulin for a short while until the body increases its insulin production again. If this is true, temporary health problems, of course, could result.

For now, the questions and risks of vanadium seem to outweigh vanadium's potential benefits, so we recommend against taking vanadium supplements unless the dose is very low or your physician recommends them. If you are diabetic and are working with a doctor who believes you would benefit from supplemental vanadium, he or she will probably advise a dose of between 25 and 100 mcg daily. Be sure to ask your doctor about bis-maltolato oxovanadium (BMOV), a newly developed, chelated form of vanadium that appears to be more biologically active and absorbable than commonly used vanadyl sulfate. The potential for toxicity of this form may be lower.

CUTTING BACK ON COPPER AND IRON

Copper and iron are both minerals essential for health, but they can pose problems for people with Syndrome X and diabetes. Excesses of either copper or iron can increase free-radical activity, and people with the high glucose levels characteristic of Syndrome X already have high levels of free radicals in their bodies. Excessive levels of copper or iron oxidize and damage tissues, age the body, and greatly increase the risk of degenerative diseases. For example, LDL cholesterol becomes an artery-blocking danger only when it oxidizes; that leaves people with a high concentration of iron or copper in their bodies at particularly heightened risk.

To promote health, adequate but not excessive amounts of bio-available copper and iron should be consumed. The best way to do this is through diet. The Anti-X diet includes good sources of copper, such as nuts and seeds, and good sources of iron, such as meats, eggs, poultry, and spinach. This should be enough copper and iron to meet most people's needs.

Many questions remain regarding copper and iron supplementation. Until more is known in this area, our recommendations are as follows:

- Avoid iron-fortified foods. White rice and white flour products are required by law to be "enriched" with supplemental iron. The iron is an inorganic form, however, that is not utilized well by the body and that may contribute to the development of iron overload (an increasingly common health problem) as well as a greater risk for heart disease.
- Avoid taking supplements of iron unless you're diagnosed with an iron deficiency or are pregnant or breast-feeding.
- If you're a premenopausal woman, and even more so if you take birth control pills, use the copper intrauterine device, or have some of the newer silver amalgam or gold alloy fillings, you should supplement with zinc but avoid taking supplements that contain copper.
- If you are pregnant or breast-feeding, particularly if you have had gestational diabetes, consult a nutritionally oriented physician to discuss whether you should take copper supplements.
- If you're a man or a postmenopausal woman, choose a supplement that has the smallest amount of copper available (no more than 2 mg per day).

The last three recommendations concerning copper come with a caveat: Make sure to have your HDL and LDL cholesterol levels monitored regularly. If you have insulin resistance and any of the other components of Syndrome X (abnormal blood fat levels, hypertension, obesity, or adult-onset diabetes), you should have your cholesterol profiles taken regularly anyway, as a way to monitor your condition. If your HDL cholesterol levels drop and your LDL cholesterol levels rise while taking zinc and little or no copper, try increasing the amount of supplemental copper you take so that you take zinc in a 15:1 ratio with copper (i.e., 30 mg zinc and 2 mg copper).

Putting This Chapter into Practice

- To prevent the development of insulin resistance and Syndrome X, it's important to avoid developing mineral deficiencies that can lead to these conditions. A multimineral supplement without iron and copper, therefore, can be helpful.

- To reverse Syndrome X, relatively high doses of chromium (1,000 mcg daily), zinc (30–50 mg daily), magnesium (400 mg), and other minerals may be needed.

CHAPTER 15

A Few More Helpful Nutrients

VIRTUALLY EVERY NUTRIENT beneficial to health also positively influences how the body deals with glucose and insulin. Some nutrients exert a direct glucose-lowering and insulin-sensitizing effect. Others are more subtle or indirect, perhaps reducing some of the characteristics of Syndrome X, such as high blood pressure or elevated cholesterol.

Done right, the Anti-X diet plan should form the foundation of your program to control Syndrome X. In addition to the nutrient supplements we have discussed, a number of other supplements may prove helpful.

In this chapter, we discuss some of these additional nutritional supplements. They can help you fine-tune your overall nutrient intake, enable your body chemistry to function a little better, and compensate for some of the undesirable foods that inevitably may creep into your diet. Consider these supplements potentially beneficial, but discretionary, depending on your individual needs.

ANTIOXIDANTS

We explained in previous chapters that alpha lipoic acid and vitamins E and C are powerful antioxidants that play important roles in controlling the symptoms and complications of Syndrome X. In addition, however, many other antioxidants, such as flavonoids and carotenoids, are important to health.

Antioxidants always work best as a team to quench disease-causing free radicals. Some antioxidants pinch-hit for others that may be low in the diet, and research by Al L. Tappel, of the University of California, Davis, has clearly shown that groups of antioxidants are more powerful than the simple sum of their parts. In experiments, Tappel has demonstrated that multiple antioxidants are better than individual antioxidants as free-radical quenchers.

It is likely that virtually every antioxidant has some positive influence on glucose and insulin, though the effects may be subtle. More clearly, antioxidants can reduce the glucose-generated free-radical damage that exacerbates diabetes, heart disease, cancer, Alzheimer's disease, and virtually every other degenerative disease. So while antioxidants may not directly or significantly counteract elevated glucose, they do control many of its consequences.

Flavonoids

It may surprise you to find that the bulk of antioxidants in foods are not vitamins or minerals. Most are members of a broad class of compounds known as polyphenols, which include the flavonoids (sometimes called bioflavonoids). Scientists have identified more than 5,000 different flavonoids in plants. Not all of them are found in edible plants, but hundreds are—and a handful of berries or a cup of green tea may contain dozens of different kinds of flavonoids.

Flavonoids aid vitamin C in shoring up the walls of blood vessels, so the walls are less permeable and don't leak blood into tissues. When blood does leak through blood-vessel walls, spontaneous bruises appear (often, people don't know how they received such bruises), and water retention and puffiness develop.

Diabetics are more likely than nondiabetics to bruise. The blood vessels of diabetics are often compromised by a combination of glucose-induced free-radical damage and a dearth of antioxidants. Diabetics are also more susceptible to eye diseases, some of which are caused by leaky blood vessels that can impair vision. Insulin resistance and Syndrome X represent the early stages of these health problems, when they can be most easily corrected.

Unfortunately, flavonoids have been relegated to second-place nutritional status, but they are highly beneficial to health, and some of them may come to be regarded as essential. Studies have found that people eating high-flavonoid diets (that is, diets rich in fruits and vegetables) have a relatively low risk of heart disease, stroke, and cancer—all diseases related, in part, to glucose problems.

In nature, flavonoids function as plant pigments. They add beautiful, appetizing colors to fruits and vegetables, making raspberries red and blueberries blue. The colors absorb and neutralize different wavelengths of light that generate free radicals when they interact with living cells. Flavonoids are plants' principal defense against free radicals. People who eat fruits and vegetables acquire the plants' free-radical-quenching benefits.

Many flavonoids have anti-inflammatory properties. These properties can be particularly helpful for people who are over-weight because obese people suffer from chronic low-grade inflammation, which increases their risk of heart disease. Of all of the antioxidants, flavonoids have the most marked anti-inflammatory effects.

For example, quercetin, a flavonoid found in onions and apples, inhibits the activity of certain molecules that promote inflammatory responses. Quercetin also has antidiabetic properties. It inhibits the activity of the enzyme aldose reductase, which promotes the formation of sorbitol, a sugar responsible for many diabetic complications.

As is the case with many other micronutrients, most people simply don't seem to consume enough flavonoids, mainly because they don't eat many fruits and vegetables. Most public-health recommendations call for people to eat five daily servings of fruits and vegetables (two of fruit, three of vegetables). Based on various surveys, however, only 9 to 32 percent of people eat this much produce, so there is no way the majority of people can obtain significant amounts of flavonoids. C. Leigh Broadhurst, a visiting scientist at the U.S. Department of Agriculture, in Beltsville, Maryland, estimates that the typical North American consumes 23 to 170 mg of flavonoids daily. It is likely that people in many other Western nations consume about the same quantity of flavonoids. Historically, humans consumed an estimated 1,000 mg daily.

Buying and Using Flavonoids

Without question, the best source of flavonoids is a diet that contains a diverse selection of vegetables and fruits. To color your diet with flavonoids, you need to look beyond iceberg lettuce for salads and potatoes as your side dish at meals. There's an old, wise saying about "eating a lot of color" for health. It referred to eating healthy, colorful foods rich in flavonoids and carotenoids (discussed in the next section). Make a point of adding colorful vegetables and fruits to your plate.

If your taste for vegetables and fruits leaves a bit to be desired, consider supplementing with some flavonoids. There are many from which to choose, including the following:

■ *Pycnogenol* is a complex of some 40 flavonoids derived from the bark of French maritime pine trees. It is, in effect, an herbal antioxidant and anti-inflammatory product. Pycnogenol helps the body maintain vitamin E and C levels, indicating that it plays a role in the antioxidant network. Therefore, it reinforces the protective effects of other antioxidants. Recent research at the University of Arizona has shown Pycnogenol to be an effective and safe anti-coagulant.

■ *Grape-seed extract,* which has been promoted as a less expensive version of Pycnogenol, is also rich in antioxidants, but its composition is somewhat different. Studies on the therapeutic benefits of Pycnogenol may not hold true for grape-seed extract.

■ *Citrus flavonoids,* found in oranges, lemons, and grapefruit, have a beneficial effect on blood-vessel walls. Considerable research has focused on their anticancer properties.

■ *Green tea,* which consists of about 30 percent flavonoids by dry weight, has cholesterol-lowering properties. One study found that men drinking nine or more cups of green tea daily had cholesterol levels about 8 mg/dl lower than that of men who drank relatively little tea. Green tea lowers cholesterol, at least partly, by reducing the absorption of dietary cholesterol. As an antioxidant flavonoid, it probably strengthens the walls of blood vessels and protects them against free-radical damage. Some research suggests that it might also lower high blood pressure, one of the symptoms of Syndrome X.

Carotenoids

More than 600 carotenoids have been identified in plants. Like the flavonoids, carotenoids are also plant pigments that do double duty as antioxidants. They make carrots orange and tomatoes red.

About 50 carotenoids show up in the Western diet, but only 14 are absorbed into the bloodstream, suggesting a biological role for them. Most research has focused on the three principal dietary carotenoids: beta-carotene, lycopene, and lutein. Of these three carotenoids, only beta-carotene can be converted to vitamin A in the body.

Of relevance to Syndrome X, beta-carotene has been shown to reduce cholesterol levels. It works by partially inhibiting the body's production of cholesterol. In one experiment, Judy A. Driskell, of the University of Nebraska, Lincoln, fed rabbits (a common model for human heart disease) a high-fat, high-cholesterol diet. She gave some of the rabbits supplements of beta-carotene, or vitamin E, or both nutrients. Beta-carotene decreased total cholesterol and LDL cholesterol levels and reduced the size of cholesterol deposits. These improvements can reduce a key symptom of Syndrome X and lower the risk of heart disease. A study of women found that approximately 9,000 IU of beta-carotene could protect against LDL oxidation, another risk factor for Syndrome X and heart disease.

Beta-carotene also activates different types of immune cells. This is important because glucose interferes with immune function, and diabetics are more susceptible to infections. It is likely that prediabetics and other people consuming large amounts of sugar have impaired immunity. While beta-carotene won't correct glucose problems, it can bolster the immune system to offset glucose-related impairments.

Buying and Using Carotenoids

The best way to obtain carotenoids, like flavonoids, is to eat a diet rich in vegetables. The problem, of course, is that most people don't. Carotenoid supplements can partly compensate. The most natural approach is a "mixed carotenoid" supplement, which sort of mimics the distribution of major carotenoids found in an assortment of foods. It's also important to know that natural beta-carotene has a different chemical structure than synthetic beta-carotene and it's a more potent antioxidant. Read labels carefully to identify the product's source. Most natural beta-carotene is derived from *D. salina* algae. If you do not see a natural source listed, assume that the product is synthetic.

Again, the health benefits of carotenoids are not directly related to the prevention or reversal of Syndrome X. However, the carotenoids (like the flavonoids) are important nutrients. If you supplement, consider taking a balanced, mixed carotenoid supplement containing natural beta- and alpha-carotene, lutein (or lutein ester), and lycopene.

Vitamin A

Vitamin A, an essential nutrient and a mild antioxidant, may benefit people with Syndrome X. In a study of 52 apparently healthy subjects, researchers noted a strong association between high vitamin A intake and insulin sensitivity. High intake of the vitamin is also associated with high levels of the protective HDL cholesterol.

It is not really clear how vitamin A influences insulin sensitivity. However, the vitamin does have hormonelike effects, and it is possible that vitamin A increases the efficiency of insulin.

Most multivitamin supplements contain vitamin A (or beta-carotene, which the body converts to vitamin A). Diabetics often have difficulty converting beta-carotene to vitamin A. Because of this, people with diabetes may need vitamin A supplements, rather than beta-carotene. If you do not take a multivitamin supplement, consider supplementing with 10,000 IU of vitamin A.

Coenzyme Q_{10}

Coenzyme Q_{10}, also known as CoQ_{10}, plays a key role in the creation of energy in cells. Secondary to this role, this vitamin-like nutrient is also an antioxidant. All cells need energy to function, and CoQ_{10} is required for efficient energy production. Of course, the fuel for most of this energy is glucose, so CoQ_{10} helps the body deal with dietary carbohydrates, the ultimate source of glucose. The discovery of this energy-promoting role of CoQ_{10} formed the basis of the 1978 Nobel Prize in chemistry. When CoQ_{10} levels are inadequate, cells cannot muster sufficient energy to perform optimally.

CoQ_{10} has a number of health benefits relative to Syndrome X. For one thing, it can prevent the free-radical oxidation of LDL cholesterol, thereby stopping an early step in the development of heart disease. A 1990s study found that patients taking daily doses of 120 mg of CoQ_{10} benefited from reductions in blood pressure and increases in protective HDL cholesterol. The researchers suggested that CoQ_{10} works by quenching free radicals and normalizing the insulin response to glucose. It can also strengthen the heart and prevent heart failure, one of the most serious of all heart diseases.

Most of the CoQ_{10} supplements sold are oil based, which means they are best absorbed with a little fat or oil. Therefore, take CoQ_{10} with a meal or a teaspoon of sugar- and salt-free almond butter or peanut butter. Some CoQ_{10} supplements are water-soluble, and these are well absorbed with or without food. CoQ_{10} is extraordinarily safe, but it is an expensive supplement. Dosages commonly range from 30 to 400 mg daily, with the higher amounts most appropriate for people with heart disease.

VITAMIN D

Vitamin D is best known for its role in aiding calcium absorption and promoting normal bone formation. There is considerable evidence, accumulated since the late 1960s, that it also plays a major role in the body's management of glucose and insulin. Vitamin D is required for the secretion of insulin by the pancreas. In experiments, vitamin D deficiency reduces the release of insulin, leading eventually to irreversible glucose intolerance.

In an article in the *British Journal of Nutrition*, B. J. Boucher of St. Bartholomew's and the Royal London Hospital Medical and Dental School, England, described vitamin D deficiency as an "avoidable risk factor" for Syndrome X and suggested that treatment of this deficiency is an important way to reduce the "worldwide epidemic" of this disorder. Some research has found that insulin resistance relates directly to low levels of vitamin D. A study of elderly Dutch men found that glucose tolerance was related to vitamin D levels, apart from other factors that might influence Syndrome X. Similarly, high blood pressure has been associated with low levels of vitamin D and calcium. Other studies have found that blood pressure is reduced with vitamin D supplements—even when there is no preexisting deficiency of the vitamin.

Although many foods (such as meat, fish, and eggs) contain vitamin D, it has been called the "sunshine vitamin" for good reason. Spending about 15 minutes or so in the sunlight stimulates the body's own production of vitamin D. There is an obvious double benefit here: If you spend some time doing physical activity outdoors, you improve your muscle tone and make vitamin D, both of which improve your glucose tolerance and insulin function.

If you don't spend much time in the sun, consider taking 400 IU of vitamin D daily. If you are taking a multivitamin supplement, you're probably already getting this amount.

GOOD FATS, BAD FATS

In earlier chapters, we discussed how the composition of dietary fats and oils has changed and suggested some ways to rebalance them. The diet should contain relatively equal amounts of the "parent" molecules of the omega-6 and omega-3 families of fats, linoleic acid and alpha-linolenic acid, respectively. Both nutrient families are needed for the normal structure and function of every cell and organ in the body. The omega-3 and omega-6 families do, however, have somewhat opposing biological properties. For example, the omega-6 fats are the building blocks for inflammatory compounds. In contrast, the omega-3 fats are the building blocks for anti-inflammatory compounds.

It is not healthy for dietary fats to be skewed one way or another. Yet because of food refining, the modern diet strongly favors the omega-6 fats. This is because, since the 1970s or so, people have been urged by public-health officials (and processed food companies) to replace saturated fats (from meat and eggs) with vegetable oils (such as soy, corn, and safflower oils). In the process, the omega-3 fats (found in fish) have virtually been squeezed out of the modern diet. People now consume 20 to 30 times more omega-6 than omega-3 fats, an imbalance that exacerbates insulin resistance and Syndrome X.

Laboratory experiments have found that animals eating diets high in saturated fats or omega-6 fats have a greater risk of developing insulin resistance. The situation is further muddied by the widespread use of partially hydrogenated trans-fatty acids in margarine and many other processed food products. Trans-fatty acids interfere with the enzyme delta-6-desaturase, needed by the body to manufacture docosahexaenoic acid (DHA), a principal omega-3 fat. Trans-fatty acids also inhibit the body's production of a very important omega-6 fat, called gamma-linolenic acid (GLA), which we discuss shortly.

Omega-3 Fats

Animal studies have shown that returning omega-3 fats back to the diet—and restoring a balance—yields many health benefits. Omega-3 fats improve glucose tolerance and can help in weight reduction, proof that the type of dietary fat is more important than the amount of fat per se. Animals that eat diets with abundant omega-3 fats gain less weight, compared with animals that eat omega-6 fats and saturated fats. Such changes may help prevent and reverse obesity, one of the hallmarks of Syndrome X. In people, omega-3 fats have been shown to reduce levels of triglycerides, a blood fat characteristic of Syndrome X and a risk factor for heart disease. Other studies have found that omega-3 fats can lower blood pressure and improve other aspects of heart function.

All in all, it's very important to maintain a balance between the omega-6 and the omega-3 fats. Because the omega-6 fats predominate in the North American diet and processed foods, you will have to take some radical action. First, as we explained in Chapter 7, cut back on vegetable oils, with the exception of extra-virgin olive oil. (Olive oil contains omega-9 fats, which are also good for health.) You'll have to read food labels carefully, because soy, corn, or safflower oil are found in nearly all processed foods. Next, make a point of adding fish to your diet at least once a week. Fish is rich in "preformed" DHA and eicosapentaenoic acid (EPA). If fish doesn't tempt your appetite, consider taking 1–3 grams of fish oils daily in capsule form.

You might also consider adding some flaxseed oil or ground flaxseed to your diet, but do so with a caveat. Many companies promote flax as a natural, vegetarian source of the omega-3 fats. It is true that flax is rich in linolenic acid, the parent molecule of DHA and EPA. However, the body must convert linolenic acid to DHA and EPA, and this conversion may be problematic in people who have consumed a lot of the omega-6 fats and trans-fatty acids. If you suffer from symptoms of Syndrome X, it is likely that your ability to handle fats has been compromised, and fish oils may provide better results.

Gamma-Linolenic Acid

It seems contradictory: People consume far too much of the omega-6 fats, but they don't get enough of one particular omega-6 fat, gamma-linolenic acid, or GLA. GLA plays numerous positive roles in health, and the human body should make it from linoleic acid, found in grains, nuts, and other foods. Unfortunately, sugar, alcohol, hydrogenated trans-fats, and diabetes interfere with the activity of delta-6-desaturase, the enzyme that plays a crucial role in converting linoleic acid to GLA.

Like other omega-6 fats and the omega-3 fats, GLA helps maintain normal nerve function. It forms part of the sheath coating the lengths of nerve cells. When these fats become unbalanced, or when overall fat levels are too low (because of zero-fat diets), these sheaths become damaged, and nerve cells don't function properly. Such nerve damage is common in diabetes and, if you recall, alpha lipoic acid and GLA are very helpful in restoring normal nerve function.

GLA can also lower cholesterol levels, and this effect is augmented when EPA is taken along with GLA. GLA works by promoting the body's production of a hormonelike prostaglandin that controls cholesterol production. Along the way, the body converts GLA to dihomo-gamma-linolenic acid (DGLA), another fatty acid that helps promote normal insulin function.

Balancing your intake of dietary fats should foster the biochemistry needed to make GLA. However, it is sometimes difficult to overcome years of eating diets high in omega-6 fats and trans-fats. For this reason, it may be desirable to take GLA supplements in the form of evening primrose oil or borage oil supplements. These supplements bypass the difficulty many people have in making GLA from linoleic acid. Typical beneficial amounts of supplemental GLA for most people range from 150 to 250 mg daily; diabetics, however, generally need up to 400 mg daily.

When taking fish-oil capsules or GLA, it is also important to take vitamin E (if you aren't already doing so). These oils are fragile and prone to free-radical damage, both on the shelf and in the body. Vitamin E can reduce this free-radical damage.

In the next chapter, we describe a number of herbal remedies that have been found helpful in preventing and treating glucose and insulin disorders. These herbs also contain many nutritional substances, such as flavonoids and carotenoids.

Putting This Chapter into Practice

- Many supplemental nutrients may help prevent insulin resistance and Syndrome X. Most of these nutrients can be obtained through the diet, a multivitamin, or individual supplements.

- To reverse Syndrome X, moderately high dosages of carotenoids, flavonoids, omega-3 fish oils, and other nutrients may be helpful.

CHAPTER 16

Herbal Remedies for Syndrome X

A FEW YEARS AGO, herbal medicines were widely perceived as unproved folk medicines, supported by many traditions but little or no science. Herbs, however, were the human race's original medicines—evidence of their medicinal use has been found with 60,000-year-old human remains. There have also been reports that primates, in the wild, seek out and use certain medicinal herbs to treat their illnesses.

Since the late 1980s, cell and molecular biologists have gained a remarkable scientific understanding of how herbal medicines work. Plants are natural pharmacies, rich in a diversity of nutrients and druglike compounds. Almost half of all modern drugs have either been developed from plant compounds or are synthetic replicas of molecules found in plants. That's a testament to the fact that herbal medicines contain biologically active molecules that influence health.

Unlike pharmaceutical drugs, which are generally built around a single, often synthetic active ingredient, herbs are extraordinarily complex chemically and can contain hundreds if not thousands of active principles. For example, more than 5,000 flavonoids and 600 carotenoids have been identified in plants. These nutrients function largely as antioxidants, but they also help regulate gene function in plants and in the animals that consume the plants. Many of these nutrients are found in common fruits and vegetables, so they have historically played a role in human nutrition and evolution. Because herbs contain very concentrated sources of these nutrients, they can often be like a natural "shot in the arm," providing a needed boost during illnesses.

Many herbs contain constituents that regulate glucose and, indirectly, insulin levels. For example, milk thistle is well known for its beneficial effects on the *liver,* an organ that interacts with the pancreas to manage the body's glucose and insulin levels. Even common culinary herbs, such as cinnamon, cloves, and bay leaves, can influence glucose levels, though more subtly, and they add spice to one's dietary life. One survey noted that more than 1,123 plants have been used in different cultures to treat diabetes. When 295 of these traditional remedies were scientifically screened, more than 81 percent turned out to have antidiabetic properties.

In this chapter, we describe some of the many herbal medicines documented for their ability to control glucose in diabetics. These herbs can also curb the progression of prediabetic conditions, such as Syndrome X. Although these medicinal herbs are remarkably safe, we recommend that you *not* use more than two of them concurrently. (In contrast, it is safe to use multiple culinary herbs because their active-ingredient concentrations are far lower than those in medicinal herbs.) Many medicinal herbs contain substances that are druglike in function, and haphazardly mixing them may occasionally be as risky as mixing too many drugs. Also, if you are a diabetic who takes insulin or hypoglycemic drugs, you should be aware that these herbs may lower your drug requirements.

SILYMARIN AND MILK THISTLE

The seeds of milk thistle (*Silybum marianum*) have been used medicinally for more than 2,000 years. They are rich in a group of powerful antioxidants known collectively as silymarin, and silymarin extracts of milk thistle are commonly sold as a concentrated source of the plant's most active ingredients.

Milk thistle has been traditionally used to treat liver-related disorders, and modern scientific research on milk thistle's silymarin extract has found it helpful in a wide range of liver disorders, including cirrhosis, viral hepatitis, and drug-induced liver disease. Substances that enhance liver function enable this organ to deal with hazardous compounds and to improve glucose control.

Many researchers attribute silymarin's benefits to its antioxidant properties. However, studies of liver cells have shown that silymarin stimulates the growth of new and healthy cells to replace those that have been damaged or destroyed.

Silymarin, Insulin Resistance, and Diabetes

In the past few years, there has been growing interest in silymarin for regulating glucose levels. In one experiment, German researchers found that silybinin (a key antioxidant constituent of silymarin) directly blocked the toxic effects of glucose on kidney cells.

The largest human study of silymarin in the treatment of diabetes yielded dramatic improvements in insulin resistance and other diabetic symptoms. This makes silymarin (and the whole milk thistle) one of the top herbs for preventing and treating Syndrome X. Mario Velussi, of Monfalcone Hospital, Goriza, Italy, asked 60 diabetics to either take 600 mg of silymarin or a placebo daily for 12 months. These were very sick patients: They had adult-onset diabetes and alcoholic cirrhosis (alcohol-induced liver damage), and they had been receiving insulin therapy for at least two years.

Although the patients' fasting glucose level rose slightly during the first month of silymarin use, it declined progressively and significantly afterward. On average, by the end of the year, fasting glucose declined from 190 mg/dl to 174 mg/dl, or by 9.5 percent; and average daily glucose dropped from 202 mg/dl to 172 mg/dl, or by 14.9 percent. These changes indicated greatly improved glucose control. Although such decreases in glucose might raise concerns about sudden bouts of *hypoglycemia* (low blood sugar), patients treated with silymarin did not experience an increase in hypoglycemic episodes, suggesting that the herbal extract worked gradually and that it stabilized glucose levels.

Patients treated with silymarin benefited in other ways, as well. Their *glucosuria* (sugar in the urine) decreased from an average of 37 grams to 22 grams daily. Glycosylated hemoglobin, a marker of diabetic control (and aging), also declined significantly. In addition, the patients' fasting insulin levels decreased by almost half— indicating a significant improvement in insulin sensitivity and reduction in insulin resistance. Meanwhile, average daily insulin requirements decreased from 55 IU to 42 IU daily. All of these changes indicated better glucose control and greater insulin sensitivity.

Two other markers showed improvement, as well. Blood levels of malondialdehyde, a marker of free-radical activity, went down. This was probably because lower glucose levels spun off fewer free radicals. In addition, levels of liver enzymes (SGOT and SGPT) dropped significantly, a sign of improved liver function.

**SILYMARIN'S EFFECTS ON INSULIN RESISTANCE
AND DIABETES**

> Glucose ↓
> Sugar in the urine ↓
> Glycosylated hemoglobin ↓
> Insulin requirements ↓
> Insulin resistance ↓
> Free-radical levels ↓
> Liver enzymes ↓

Supplementing with Silymarin

Silymarin and milk thistle are among the most popular herbal supplements sold in health-food stores. A survey of patients at a *hepatology* (liver) clinic associated with Oregon Health Sciences University, Portland, found that many of them were using silymarin or milk thistle, in addition to their prescribed medications, and half of those patients felt that silymarin helped reduce their symptoms.

Stresses to the liver make it work harder and take a toll on the liver's production of antioxidants, such as glutathione, and its ability to regulate glucose. These stresses include exposures to a wide variety of synthetic chemicals, from air pollution to alcohol. By bolstering liver function, silymarin can maintain normal liver function, so the organ does its job better.

As with most herbs, the dosage must be individualized, though silymarin appears safe even at high dosages. Velussi's study with diabetics used 600 mg of silymarin daily (without any other type of supplementation). Unless you're diabetic, you probably don't need that much. If you have signs of Syndrome X, consider starting at a lower dose, such as 200 mg daily.

As with many herbal products on the market, silymarin comes in standardized and nonstandardized formulations. Although these products are different, both are good, provided that they are produced by reputable companies. A standardized product is advantageous in that it contains a defined amount of silymarin, such as 140 mg per capsule. The disadvantage is that the refining or extraction process may eliminate smaller, synergistic constituents that also have medicinal value. Standardized products also cost more than nonstandardized ones. Nature's Way makes an excellent standardized silymarin supplement called Thisilyn.

This does not mean that nonstandardized products are bad. Nonstandardized products have the advantage of containing more whole-herb constituents, due to less processing of the herb. Many herbalists prefer this broader range of ingredients because they have a greater natural synergy than more refined products. For example, A. Vogel Bioforce, a Swiss-based company, markets an excellent milk-thistle-complex tincture that is very consistent in potency from batch to batch. We encourage you to experiment a little in order to find the silymarin or milk-thistle product that works best for you.

THE TOP HERBS FOR CONTROLLING GLUCOSE, INSULIN RESISTANCE, AND SYNDROME X

Milk thistle (silymarin extract)
Bitter melon
Fenugreek
Gymnema sylvestre (gurmar)
Garlic

BITTER MELON

Bitter melon (*Momordica charantia*), also known as bitter gourd, balsam pear, and karela, is technically a fruit, not an herb. It is commonly sold in Asian grocery stores and has impressive glucose-lowering effects. Bitter melon can be consumed as a side dish (like squash), a juice, or a decoction, and it is also available in supplement form. (We explain how to make a decoction in the following section.) The active ingredients are a number of glucose-lowering compounds and an insulin-like protein. Bitter melon improves glucose tolerance and can reduce symptoms of Syndrome X and diabetes.

Both animal and human studies have demonstrated the benefits of bitter melon. In one experiment with healthy laboratory rats, glucose levels decreased by 10–15 percent one hour after being given bitter-melon extract; in diabetic rats, glucose dropped by 26 percent after three and a half hours. Bitter melon appeared to work by improving the utilization of glucose, not by increasing the secretion of insulin. Another study with rats found that bitter melon reduced glucose levels by half in diabetic rats. In addition, animals with lower glucose levels were less likely to develop diabetic cataracts.

In a small clinical trial, researchers gave six adult-onset diabetic patients a 200-milliliter (ml) decoction of bitter melon, an amount comparable to 3.3 ounces, once a day for three weeks. Fasting glucose declined by 54 percent after three weeks, and after seven weeks, all subjects' glucose levels were near normal! Numerous other trials, most conducted in India and Pakistan, have shown similar benefits. In one study, 18 newly diagnosed adult-onset diabetics received 100 ml (one-tenth of a liter, or about 1.6 ounces) of the fresh juice of unripe bitter melon. Three fourths of the patients experienced significant improvements in glucose tolerance.

How to Use Bitter Melon

Use the *unripe*, not the ripe, bitter melon to treat elevated glucose and diabetes. Fresh juices or decoctions are often the preferred forms of bitter melon. You can make a decoction by finely chopping the fruit, then pouring boiling water over it. Next, steep and strain it, and let it cool. Drink one six-ounce glass daily. To improve its flavor, mix in a little cinnamon powder.

You can also cook sliced bitter melon and eat it as a side dish with one or two meals daily. Try baking it like squash, or slicing and cooking it in a skillet with olive oil. Again, use the unripe fruit.

If you prefer supplements to the fruit, you can purchase bitter-melon supplements at many health-food stores. One such product, made by the Eclectic Institute (see the appendix), contains freeze-dried bitter melon. Another product, made by Nature's Way and called "Blood Sugar," contains bitter melon, fenugreek, *Gymnema sylvestre*, nopal leaves, and other nutrients that help regulate glucose levels.

FENUGREEK

Fenugreek seeds (*Trigonella foenum-graecum*) have a long history of use in Indian cooking and in Ayurvedic medicine for the treatment of diabetes and heart disease. Scientific studies have shown that fenugreek-seed powder can lower glucose levels and improve a person's cholesterol profile. The seeds are about 50 percent fiber, which slows digestion and the postmeal rise in glucose.

Fenugreek-seed powder, in a wide range of dosages, has been shown to lower glucose levels in diabetic patients. In one study, researchers gave patients with heart disease and/or diabetes 2.5 grams of fenugreek-seed powder twice daily for three months. In patients with both heart disease and diabetes, total cholesterol and triglyceride levels decreased significantly. In patients with relatively mild diabetes, fenugreek significantly reduced both fasting and postmeal glucose levels. More seriously ill diabetics were helped only slightly, and healthy subjects experienced no change in glucose levels.

Another study involved adding 100 grams of powdered fenugreek seeds to the daily meals of 10 diabetic patients. After 10 days, the added fenugreek reduced fasting blood-sugar levels and improved the patients' responses to glucose tolerance tests. The urinary excretion of glucose decreased by 54 percent, a sign of much better glucose metabolism, and total cholesterol and LDL cholesterol levels were also lowered. These are all changes that can help reverse Syndrome X.

To demonstrate the herb's cholesterol-lowering properties, researchers placed 89 subjects on a low-fat diet for 12 weeks, then gave them supplemental fenugreek-seed powder (60 grams/day) for another 12 weeks. Compared with people getting a placebo, those consuming the fenugreek-seed powder had a 13 percent decrease in overall cholesterol and a 15 percent reduction in LDL cholesterol levels. Furthermore, the fenugreek seeds increased HDL levels by 6 percent.

How to Use Fenugreek

Fenugreek-seed powder is sold in bulk form in most Indian grocery stories. If you have a choice of fenugreek products, opt for the defatted and debitterized powder. You can add some of it to foods you prepare (such as meat loafs), but you might find more interesting recipes in an Indian cookbook. At high doses, fenugreek-seed powder can cause flatulence. If this happens, reduce the dose.

Some researchers, such as C. Leigh Broadhurst, recommend mixing a small amount of fenugreek-seed powder (one quarter to one full teaspoon) in a glass of water. The taste leaves a lot to be desired, but it can be improved by adding a cinnamon stick as a natural flavor enhancer. Follow the same approach when making fenugreek tea.

Standardized fenugreek capsules are now on the market. To improve glucose control and lower cholesterol levels, take supplements containing 5–10 grams of fenugreek extract daily.

GYMNEMA SYLVESTRE

Gymnema sylvestre, also known as gurmar, is another herb from India's Ayurvedic medical traditions that has been used for centuries to neutralize excess sugar. As with many other Ayurvedic herbs, its properties have been confirmed by scientific studies. Some research in insulin-dependent diabetics has found that it can increase insulin secretion by the pancreas. Other research indicates that it can increase the efficiency of insulin in reducing glucose levels.

In one study, 22 adult diabetics taking glucose-lowering drugs were also given *Gymnema* leaf extracts. All of the patients benefited from significant reductions in glucose and glycosylated hemoglobin after taking *Gymnema* for 18 months. In fact, 5 of the patients were able to safely discontinue taking their glucose-reducing drugs as long as they kept taking *Gymnema*. The subjects reported that they were more alert, less exhausted, and had an overall better sense of well-being.

Some research indicates that *Gymnema* promotes the regeneration of pancreatic beta cells, which produce insulin. If so, *Gymnema* would be of considerable benefit in people with either juvenile- or adult-onset diabetes. Positive responses in a couple of diabetic patients prompted Indian researchers to more rigorously test *Gymnema* on laboratory rats. They found that *Gymnema* supplementation resulted in a near-normal fasting and postmeal glucose response.

A similar experiment on 27 insulin-dependent diabetics also had positive results. Glucose levels declined, and insulin requirements were reduced during the yearlong study. Glycosylated hemoglobin levels were also reduced. Some of the subjects had an improvement in neuropathic symptoms, evidenced by reduced pain in arms and legs, within a couple weeks of taking gurmar. Several patients also described an improved sense of physical well-being and greater mental sharpness.

How to Use Gymnema sylvestre

Gymnema is very bitter tasting. We therefore recommend the supplements. To help in glucose tolerance and insulin resistance, take 75–150 mg of standardized *Gymnema sylvestre* extract daily.

GARLIC

Not all herbs have mysterious origins or unfamiliar flavors. People are often surprised that garlic (*Allium sativum*) possesses powerful medicinal properties. This common food has a modest effect on glucose levels, but a much more significant and consistent effect on cholesterol and triglyceride levels. Onions, a close relative, contain some of the same active ingredients, but in much lower concentrations.

One of the difficulties with interpreting garlic research is that findings are occasionally contradictory. Some studies find that garlic reduces glucose; others do not. Similarly, some studies show it to reduce cholesterol and triglycerides; again, others do not. These contradictions might be explained, in part, by the many different forms of garlic used in these studies. Some researchers use raw garlic or garlic oil. Other scientists, with support from makers of garlic supplements, use different types of supplements. We believe that the different methods used to process garlic for supplements select for a different spectrum of compounds, which have slightly different properties.

All garlic is rich in sulfur, a key nutritional building block for the body. However, a clove of garlic is relatively inert until it is sliced, diced, or cooked. When a clove is damaged in one of these ways, it reacts with oxygen and begins forming dozens of new sulfur compounds. These compounds donate large amounts of sulfur-containing amino acids and other sulfur-containing chemicals to myriad biochemical reactions in the body. Perhaps not surprisingly, studies have found that virtually every form of garlic, including the garlic powder sold in supermarkets, has some beneficial effects. However, the potency of garlic will vary somewhat among products, and freshly prepared garlic and supplements seem to be the most biologically active.

Garlic and Glucose Control

Garlic can sometimes lower glucose levels. For example, a German study found that daily consumption of 800 mg of garlic powder reduced glucose levels by 11.6 percent over four weeks. The subjects' glucose levels, which were in the normal range to start, dropped from an average of 89.4 mg/dl to 79 mg/dl. Similar findings have been reported in animal studies. Unfortunately, research on garlic's glucose-lowering properties is not consistent, and most studies have found it *not* to have an effect on glucose. However, garlic does have other benefits relevant to Syndrome X.

Garlic Benefits the Cardiovascular System

Although garlic's role in reducing glucose levels may not always be consistent, there is strong evidence that it can reduce cholesterol and triglyceride levels, as well as other risk factors for heart disease.

This is important because Syndrome X greatly increases the risk of heart disease.

The evidence in favor of garlic's cholesterol-lowering properties is very strong. Two comprehensive analyses of garlic studies found that supplements reduced cholesterol levels by an average of 9–12 percent. In a typical study, Adesh K. Jain, of Tulane University School of Medicine, New Orleans, gave either daily garlic supplements (900 mg of the Kwai brand) or a placebo to 42 healthy men and women with moderately elevated cholesterol levels. After 12 weeks, subjects taking garlic supplements had a 6 percent drop in total cholesterol levels and an 11 percent decrease in LDL. People taking the placebo had only slight improvements.

Similarly, Manfred Steiner, of East Carolina University, Greenville, North Carolina, gave a different brand of garlic supplements (7.2 grams of Kyolic aged garlic extract) to 41 men with moderately high cholesterol levels. After six months, men taking the garlic supplements had reductions of 7 percent in total cholesterol and 4.6 percent in LDL. The subjects also benefited from a 5.5 percent decline in *systolic blood pressure* (the first, higher number in a blood-pressure reading).

Garlic also functions as a natural blood thinner by reducing the body's production of thromboxane compounds, which stimulate blood clotting. In a study of male subjects, researchers documented that eating one clove of fresh garlic daily for 16 weeks reduced thromboxane levels by 80 percent and cholesterol by 20 percent.

German researchers demonstrated garlic's anticlotting properties in a study of patients with *peripheral artery occlusive disease,* a condition characterized by blood clots in the legs. Doctors encourage patients with this disorder to walk because increased blood flow reduces the likelihood of clot formation. However, walking typically becomes painful after a short distance, and this discourages patients from physical activity.

The researchers gave 64 patients with peripheral artery occlusive disease either a placebo or 800 mg of garlic powder supplements daily for 12 weeks. During the course of the study, patients taking garlic supplements were able to walk about one third farther without pain, compared with those taking the placebo.

The same researchers also noted that garlic's hypertension-reducing effects could be detected after patients took a *single* garlic-powder capsule. The reason may be that garlic contains a natural *ACE inhibitor,* which works somewhat like prescription drugs that block the body's production of an enzyme involved in hypertension. The difference is that garlic's natural ACE inhibitor occurs at a low dose and is safe.

How to Use Garlic

Our first recommendation is simple: Add lots of garlic to your food. It is one of the few medicinal herbs that is potent, inexpensive, *and* tasty. Ignore supplement ads that discourage you from eating fresh or cooked garlic because it might upset your stomach. Most people tolerate garlic very well.

If you hate the odor of garlic or find that it does upset your stomach, then consider taking a supplement. The major brands are Kyolic, Kwai, Pure-Gar, and Garlicin. Each has its advocates, studies, and advertising campaigns, and because of different preparation methods, each of these products probably contains a slightly different spectrum of compounds and has somewhat different effects. However, all of these supplements are probably beneficial. Most of the studies show a cholesterol-lowering effect at 800–900 mg daily, and this may add up (depending on the brand) to several capsules daily. If you are taking garlic with other supplements, you can certainly get by with a much lower dose.

The only caution related to garlic is that its blood-thinning effect could amplify that of other anticoagulants, including the drug warfarin, aspirin, vitamin E, and ginkgo biloba. If you decide to increase your intake of garlic or to take garlic supplements, consider decreasing your intake of other anticoagulants. If you are taking a prescription anticoagulant, discuss your medications—pharmaceutical or natural—with a physician who understands their interactions.

OTHER HERBS OF VALUE IN SYNDROME X

A great many herbs have been shown to improve glucose tolerance and insulin sensitivity. The fact that diabetics and other people with glucose disorders so often respond favorably to herbal medicines indicates that they may have been lacking some important nutrients. What follows are brief discussions of other herbs found to have some glucose-lowering effects.

Green and Black Teas

Teas are rich in antioxidant polyphenols and flavonoids, and many studies have found this beverage (or its extracts) to reduce the risk of heart disease and cancer. *Green tea,* a common beverage in China, is made from unfermented leaves. *Black tea,* preferred in Western nations, is made by fermenting green tea. A recent study by researchers at Nanchang University, China, found that both teas can reduce glucose and triglyceride levels.

The researchers fed 12-month-old laboratory rats either green and black teas (as part of their diets or in their drinking water) or a standard diet and plain water. These 1-year-old rats were physiologically similar to 50-year-old men. Green tea reduced glucose levels by almost 24 percent and triglycerides by 33 percent. Black tea was almost as good, reducing glucose by 23 percent and triglycerides by 25 percent.

Large sugar molecules, called polysaccharides, in tea may inhibit the absorption of glucose, according to the researchers. Another tea compound, diphenylamine, appears to promote the burning of glucose.

Nopal

Nopal, from the prickly pear cactus (*Opuntia ficus, Opuntia strepacantha*), is a traditional Mexican folk remedy for diabetes. Some studies show that nopal capsules can significantly lower both glucose and insulin levels in diabetics. Others have found that nopal does not lower glucose, but that it prevents a rise in glucose levels following the consumption of refined sugars.

Nopal's benefits are offset by the quantities required for a glucose-lowering effect. In many of the studies, patients took 30 capsules per day, which reduces the practicality of nopal supplements. However, as part of a broader dietary or supplement program, nopal can probably help reduce glucose levels. Nopal is available in cans in Mexican grocery stores.

Colosolic Acid

Colosolic acid, known also as Regulin, is an extract of the leaves of *Lagerstroemia specious L.,* a Philippine plant. Filipino and Japanese scientists have researched its effect on glucose levels, and it is a promising herbal supplement.

Colosolic acid has an insulin-like effect and has been described as a "phyto-insulin." Both animal studies and human trials have found it to be safe and effective in lowering glucose levels. It has an advantage over insulin, in that it can be taken orally, whereas insulin must be injected.

A Japanese study, conducted in 1998, tested colosolic acid on 23 subjects with glucose levels of 110 mg/dl, which is at the high end of the normal range. The subjects received either a placebo or three standardized 25 mg Regulin tablets three times daily (after meals) for four weeks. The total daily dose of colosolic acid was 0.16 mg, or 160 mcg. Glucose levels declined in most patients.

Stevia

Stevia, an extract of *Stevia rebaudiana*, plays two roles in curbing glucose disorders. First, it has modest glucose-lowering properties. Second, it is extremely sweet and has gained a following as a natural alternative to sugar and other caloric sweeteners.

In a Brazilian study, researchers gave 16 healthy subjects extracts of 5 grams of stevia leaves at six-hour intervals for three days. The subjects were given glucose tolerance tests (roughly the equivalent of a soft drink and a couple of doughnuts), and their responses were compared with subjects given only the glucose tolerance tests. The stevia extracts significantly decreased glucose levels during the test and after awakening in the morning.

Stevia is also 200–300 times sweeter than sugar. In other words, a little bit goes a long way. In Japan, stevia sales reportedly account for about half of all commercial sweeteners. In the United States, the Food and Drug Administration (FDA) has tried to limit the importation, distribution, and sale of stevia—going so far as to even try to destroy books on this natural sweetener. The FDA does seem to be on an antistevia campaign. Could the agency be helping industry to keep a competing sweetener off the market? That's what many stevia advocates believe.

Despite the political situation, stevia is sold in health-food stores in dry-leaf form, white stevia powder, and water- and alcohol-based extracts. It doesn't make much sense to trade off sugar for alcohol, so we recommend the water-based stevia extracts or the white extract powder. It's best to train your taste buds away from the sweet taste, but when you do have the desire for sweetness without the harmful consequences associated with sugar, using stevia is your best choice. To learn about how to order stevia and how to use stevia in food and drinks, refer to Appendix A.

Holy Basil

Though related to common basil, holy basil (*Ocimum sanctum*) is a different species. Animal experiments have found that its leaves can reduce fasting and postmeal glucose levels. An Indian study of 17 diabetics found that 1 gram of holy basil leaf reduced fasting glucose levels by 20.8 percent. In addition, cholesterol levels went down by 11 percent and triglyceride by 16 percent.

Culinary Herbs and Spices

If you have needed an excuse to use less salt and pepper and to increase your use of more flavorful culinary herbs and spices, consider their glucose-lowering properties. Laboratory experiments by U.S. Department of Agriculture researchers have found that cinnamon, cloves, and bay leaves can greatly improve insulin sensitivity. Another study found that coriander can reduce glucose levels.

Culinary herbs and spices are rich sources of antioxidants. Think of them as tasty sources of some of the nutrients found in salads, plus some. Recent studies have found oregano and rosemary to contain powerful antioxidants. They probably also help control glucose levels, though this hasn't been proved yet.

Rather than search for these herbs and spices in the supplement department, simply add them to foods you bake, such as chicken. A pinch here and there contributes to your overall dietary fortification against insulin resistance and Syndrome X.

Many herbal remedies can prevent Syndrome X, just as can vitamin and mineral supplements, physical activity, and dietary improvements. All of these approaches work best when combined into a broad health program. In the next and final chapter, we provide you with some guidelines for adapting this information to your personal needs.

Putting This Chapter into Practice

- To prevent insulin resistance and Syndrome X, emphasize culinary herbs, such as garlic, cinnamon, cloves, and bay leaves. If there are family risk factors for these disorders, take silymarin or milk-thistle supplements as well.

- To reverse insulin resistance and Syndrome X, take silymarin or milk-thistle supplements. In addition, however, experiment with some of the other herbs, one at a time, to determine whether they may also help.

PART FOUR

Individualizing Your Anti-X Program

CHAPTER 17

Customizing for Your Personal Needs

By READING THIS BOOK, you've learned that Syndrome X is a nutritional disease of our modern times. It is increasingly prevalent but can be prevented and reversed through a rational diet, moderate physical activity, and the selective use of supplements.

In this final chapter, we describe how to apply what you have learned in this book in practical terms. We offer various templates to follow in adapting our diet, physical activity, and supplement recommendations to your individual requirements.

It is important to note, however, that just as one shoe does not fit all people, these templates may not exactly fit your needs. It would be impossible to develop a handful of guidelines that map to the specific requirements of every imaginable person. These templates should be viewed as a starting point, but certainly not the last word, in your Anti-X program. Bear in mind several key points as you apply our dietary, physical activity, and supplement recommendations:

IT'S BETTER TO TAKE SMALL STEPS THAN NONE AT ALL. You may feel overwhelmed when trying to change your diet, physical activity patterns, and supplements all at once. Although a combination of these three Anti-X components will produce the greatest benefits, we realize that you may not be able to change your life in a day, or a week. So start somewhere, such as by incorporating some of our Anti-X meals, going for short walks, and taking a multivitamin supplement. When these changes start to feel second-nature to you, gradually build on them to get more benefits.

233

STAY FLEXIBLE, AND EXPERIMENT A LITTLE. This is the only way you can really determine what works best for you. No diet or supplement plan should be so rigid that it starts to resemble a religious ritual. Be willing to increase or lower the dose of some supplements within a reasonable range. As an example, alpha lipoic acid functions as an excellent antioxidant at 50 mg daily, but 200–300 mg or more daily may be needed to significantly lower glucose or increase insulin function.

RECOGNIZE THAT BODIES CHANGE WITH TIME AND THAT DIET, PHYSICAL ACTIVITY, AND SUPPLEMENTS MUST EVOLVE ACCORDINGLY. The plan that works for you this year may have to be modified somewhat by next year. Pay close attention to how you feel and to various indicators of your health, including the size of your waistline; your glucose, cholesterol, and triglyceride levels; your blood pressure; and your overall energy levels and physical stamina.

TRUST YOUR INTUITION. At this point, you have learned a lot about diet and how some individual nutrients function. In many respects, you are the best judge of your health, and you may intuit which supplements may be best suited for you. For example, you may feel that, given your health, alpha lipoic acid may be the best supplement to complement your Anti-X diet. On the other hand, you may get a strong sense that silymarin, which has many similar benefits, is better for you. Listen to your gut feelings.

THE DIET RECOMMENDATIONS IN THIS BOOK ARE EXTRAORDINARILY SAFE. Human beings evolved eating a diet high in animal protein, vegetables, and vitamins and minerals—*not* high in sugars and other refined carbohydrates. In essence, our diet recommendations resemble those best suited, biologically, for human beings.

THE NUTRITIONAL SUPPLEMENTS ARE SAFE AT THE DOSAGES WE RECOMMEND. Unlike prescription drugs, vitamins and minerals play normal roles in health, and they have a wide margin of safety. Similarly, herbal remedies are safe when taken individually or combined with just one or two other herbs. However, as we noted in Chapter 16, because herbal medicines sometimes have druglike side effects, there may be some risk of side effects if you take more than a couple of the herbal remedies simultaneously. A naturopathic physician (N.D.) skilled in herbal medicine can guide you more specifically about safe and suitable combinations.

MODERATE PHYSICAL ACTIVITY IS VITAL FOR BOTH PREVENTING AND REVERSING INSULIN RESISTANCE, SYNDROME X, OBESITY, AND TYPE 2 DIABETES. It doesn't matter how you become and stay active, just that you do. In the templates that follow, we offer some suggestions for physical activity under each heading, but our suggestions certainly don't mean that the types of exercise mentioned are helpful only for that physical condition. They're simply ideas. Any type of physical activity you like and do regularly offers benefits. As you're reading along, take note of the suggestions that seem most fun and doable for you, and refer back to the more comprehensive suggestions we offer in Chapter 9. Then put these ideas into practice. The more active you are, the more you'll move yourself away from insulin resistance and all its accompanying health consequences.

LIMIT YOUR INTAKE OF ALCOHOLIC BEVERAGES. Although we have focused chiefly on diet, physical activity, and supplements, it is of paramount importance that you limit your intake of alcoholic beverages (especially beer and hard liquor) and that you not use tobacco products.

YOUR RESPONSE TO THE DIET AND SUPPLEMENTS WILL VARY, DEPENDING ON A NUMBER OF FACTORS. It will be influenced by your current health, how well you follow the diet, how regularly you take the supplements, and your level of physical activity. If you follow our recommendations closely, there is a good chance that you will notice improvements in how you feel in less than a week, but other changes may take several weeks or months. During this time, your glucose, blood fats, and blood pressure should start to normalize.

YOU ARE UNDER AGE 35, IN GOOD HEALTH, AND OF NORMAL WEIGHT . . .

If you are young and in good health, you should be guided by the desire to maintain your health and prevent disease. Aging is inevitable, and with it comes a decreasing efficiency in how your body processes nutrients—and a greater risk of Syndrome X. You can take an active role in maintaining your health by limiting your intake of refined carbohydrates, engaging in regular physical activity, and taking some supplements.

Diet Recommendations

Follow the Basic Anti-X Diet Plan. Read food labels, and become more discriminating about what you eat in restaurants, snack on, and buy in supermarkets.

Physical Activity

Make a point of including some physical activities in your life. Enjoy a walk, ride a bike, or go swimming several times a week. You can certainly exercise more intensively, but you don't have to.

Recommended Daily Supplements

- A solid once-a-day type supplement, such as AlphaBetic (see Appendix A for more details)
- An "antioxidant formula" that contains several antioxidants, including 400 IU of natural vitamin E

YOU ARE OVER AGE 35, IN GOOD HEALTH, AND OF NORMAL WEIGHT . . .

Around the age of 35, many people start to get a sense of their individual mortality. Between 35 and 45, they may start developing some borderline symptoms of Syndrome X, such as moderately elevated cholesterol and blood pressure, as well as a few unwanted pounds in the midsection. If this sounds like you, keep in mind that it is easier to reverse these symptoms now than it will be in a few years.

Diet Recommendations

Follow the Basic Anti-X Diet Plan but, at your discretion, add some of the menu plans and recipes from the Anti-X Extra-Healing Diet Plan. Develop Anti-X consumer savvy, and apply it in restaurants and supermarkets to keep yourself healthy.

Physical Activity

Frequently incorporate small amounts of physical activity into your lifestyle, and do it in creative ways. Some suggestions: Do yardwork. Take moonlight walks with your significant other. Dance the night away every so often, or play regular games of golf.

Recommended Daily Supplements

- High-potency multivitamin
- Multimineral supplement (without iron and copper)
- High-potency antioxidant supplement (Your total intake of vitamin E should be around 400 IU; vitamin C, 500–1,000 mg; and alpha lipoic acid, 50 mg.)

YOU ARE IN GOOD HEALTH BUT HAVE FAMILY RISK FACTORS FOR DIABETES OR HEART DISEASE . . .

Having family members (e.g., parents or siblings) with adult-onset diabetes or heart disease increases your risk of developing these diseases. The reason may be a genetic propensity, or simply that you have shared the same unhealthy eating habits. Often underlying a familial risk of diabetes or heart disease are risk factors for Syndrome X. As incredible as it might sound, a good diet and the right combination of supplements can often compensate for some genetic weaknesses (because they provide the nutrients to help weak genes function better). You can reduce your risk by improving your eating habits, becoming a little more active physically, and taking some supplements.

Diet Recommendations

Follow the Basic Anti-X Diet Plan.

Physical Activity

Physical activity is more important for you than for someone in good health who doesn't have family risk factors for diabetes and heart disease. Begin by going for walks during lunch, and walking down a couple flights of stairs instead of taking the elevator. Also try taking a bike for occasional spins around your neighborhood.

Recommended Daily Supplements

- Either AlphaBetic or a high-potency multivitamin/multimineral supplement (preferably without iron and copper)
- An additional antioxidant formula so that your intake of vitamin E is approximately 400 IU; vitamin C, 500–1,000 mg; and alpha lipoic acid, 100 mg

YOU HAVE CRAVINGS FOR CARBOHYDRATES . . .

Carbohydrate cravings (e.g., for pastas, breads, chocolates) are almost always a sign that you are not eating enough protein. They typically indicate some form of glucose intolerance, which places you on the path to insulin resistance and Syndrome X. Take carbohydrate cravings as early warning signs that your diet or stress level is out of balance and that it's time to make lifestyle changes to enhance your health.

Diet Recommendations

To reduce your cravings for carbohydrates, reduce your intake of grains, starchy vegetables, and sweets, and increase your consumption of protein. Don't be afraid of eating too much protein; be more concerned about eating too little. To hold cravings at bay, you need to eat an amount of protein that might seem like a lot, compared to what you're used to eating.

Avoiding refined carbohydrates might be difficult for the first week, but your cravings should decrease considerably after this time. When you have a sweet tooth, try sucking on a cinnamon stick.

Follow the Basic Anti-X Diet Plan, but be sure to avoid wheat; it's a common trigger to cravings. If you try all these suggestions and still crave carbohydrates, switch to the Anti-X Extra-Healing Diet Plan for several weeks.

Physical Activity

Manage stress effectively by taking regular minibreaks of physical activity. Take a short, brisk walk in the morning. Turn on your favorite music, and dance to the beat. Take yourself shopping, and walk from one end of the mall to the other.

Recommended Daily Supplements

- Take AlphaBetic multivitamin/multimineral supplement.
- Add chromium, so your total intake is 400–500 mcg.
- Add zinc, so your total intake is 30 mg.
- Optional: Add alpha lipoic acid, so your total intake is 100 mg.
- Optional: Add silymarin or milk-thistle complex, following label instructions for daily use.

YOU HAVE ELEVATED GLUCOSE . . .

Elevated levels of fasting glucose, ranging from high normal to pre-diabetic (110–140 mg/dl), indicate that you are eating too many sugars and other refined carbohydrates. High glucose levels also indicate that you are probably insulin resistant, as well. You can, however, improve your glucose tolerance and reduce insulin resistance in just one day. The key is to eat a high-protein, low-carbohydrate breakfast, and then emphasize small amounts of protein in regular amounts throughout the rest of the day.

Diet Recommendations

Follow the Anti-X Extra-Healing Diet Plan for a couple of months or until your fasting glucose falls in the 80–100 mg/dl range. After your glucose levels normalize, switch to the Basic Anti-X Diet Plan.

Physical Activity

The more muscle you have, the more efficiently your body burns glucose (and gets rid of it). One low-stress resistance activity that builds muscle is swimming—or just splashing around in a pool. Other resistance activities include pushing a baby in a stroller and mowing the lawn. Dancing is a great way to work your muscles and burn up glucose while having a lot of fun.

Recommended Daily Supplements

Your supplements should be geared to reducing glucose levels, improving insulin action, and counteracting the effects of glucose-generated free radicals.

- Build your supplement program around AlphaBetic.
- Add extra alpha lipoic acid, so you're taking 200–300 mg.
- Add extra chromium, so you're taking 400–1,000 mcg.
- Add extra zinc, so you're taking 15–30 mg.
- Optional: For added protection against heart disease and other degenerative diseases, add extra vitamin E, so you're taking 400–500 IU, and extra vitamin C, so you're taking around 1,000 mg per day.
- Optional: Try Nature's Way "Blood Sugar" supplement, which contains several glucose-lowering herbs.

YOU HAVE INSULIN RESISTANCE (WITH OR WITHOUT HIGH GLUCOSE) . . .

Insulin resistance typically builds up slowly over a number of years, and it can often mask the glucose-boosting effect of sugars and other carbohydrates. Insulin resistance, the cornerstone of Syndrome X, is the result of your body overproducing insulin and your glucose-burning muscle cells becoming insensitive to the hormone. It's relatively easy, though, to reduce insulin resistance and improve insulin function.

Diet Recommendations

Try sprinkling cinnamon on many different types of foods—oatmeal, baked sweet potatoes, apples, and even in coffee. Look for new recipes you can try that use cinnamon, cloves, and bay leaves. If your weight is normal, follow the Basic Anti-X Diet Plan. If you are overweight, even a little, follow the Anti-X Extra-Healing Diet Plan.

Physical Activity

Make a conscious effort to become a little more physical. Go for walks and bicycle rides. Make your bicycle ride enjoyable, and resist the temptation to be competitive. Try gardening—growing vegetables or flowers—so you can work with the earth and enjoy the great outdoors.

Recommended Daily Supplements

- Build your supplement regimen around AlphaBetic.
- Add additional alpha lipoic acid, so you are taking 200–300 mg.
- Add additional chromium, so you are taking 400–1,000 mcg.
- Add additional zinc, so you are taking 30 mg.
- Add additional magnesium, so you are taking 400 mg.
- Optional: Add 140–200 mg of silymarin.

YOU HAVE HYPERTENSION . . .

Elevated blood pressure is often the result of excessive insulin, and hypertensive people are commonly insulin resistant. You can reduce blood pressure by improving insulin function and by improving blood-vessel function.

Diet Recommendations

If you are overweight, follow the Anti-X Extra-Healing Diet Plan. Eat as many fresh foods as possible, and try to choose canned or packaged foods low in sodium (containing less than 140 mg sodium per serving, as listed on the "Nutrition Facts" label of the product). Use garlic liberally in the foods you make, and eat cold-water fish (such as salmon, trout, or tuna) at least 1–2 times weekly.

Eating four stalks of celery daily is another blood-pressure-reducing strategy to try. The vegetable contains 3-n-butyl phthalide, a blood-pressure-lowering compound. If celery by itself seems boring, try snacking on it with some of the cottage cheese spreads described in Chapter 8, or with almond butter or peanut butter, or with sugar-free, olive-oil-based salad dressings. Also add celery in cooking and to various salads. For convenience, keep a few cut stalks in a glass of water in the refrigerator so you have easy-to-grab celery sticks for snacking.

Physical Activity

Stick with moderate physical activities, such as walking, light swimming, housework, or gardening. Keep things fun, and gradually incorporate more activity into your life.

Recommended Daily Supplements

- A high-potency multivitamin supplement
- A multimineral supplement without iron or copper
- Magnesium intake of about 400 mg
- About 1–3 grams of omega-3 fish-oil capsules

YOU ARE 10–20 POUNDS OVERWEIGHT . . .

Your weight can creep up with you hardly noticing it, as can your risk of developing disease. Obesity increases your risk of heart disease, diabetes, and possibly cancer. Keep in mind that insulin promotes the storage of fat, and being overweight is a sign of excess insulin. Abdominal fat especially is one of the key indicators of Syndrome X. So, if your waist size is a few inches more than it was a decade ago, you are probably insulin resistant and heading toward Syndrome X. You can reverse this process relatively easily, though, by making positive lifestyle changes.

Diet Recommendations

Try the Basic Anti-X Diet Plan for two months, but be sure to avoid wheat products, which are common triggers to overeating for many people. If you lose 5–10 pounds during this time, stick with the diet. If you are unable to lose that much weight, shift to the Anti-X Extra-Healing Diet Plan. After you lose the weight, gradually return to the Basic Anti-X Diet Plan.

Physical Activity

Find a walking partner (coworker or spouse), and walk for a few blocks after lunch or dinner. As your stamina increases, walk farther and faster: You'll find yourself walking away the pounds.

Recommended Daily Supplements

Supplements that help burn glucose and improve insulin function won't help you lose weight by themselves, but combined with a low-carbohydrate diet and physical activity, they can greatly improve the efficiency of how your body deals with carbohydrate calories.

- A once-a-day multivitamin/multimineral supplement without iron or copper, such as AlphaBetic
- Alpha lipoic acid, so you are taking a total of 50–200 mg
- Chromium, so you are taking a total of 400–800 mcg

YOU ARE MORE THAN 20 POUNDS OVERWEIGHT . . .

If you are more than 20 pounds overweight, you have a significantly greater risk of developing heart disease and diabetes—or both. This degree of obesity indicates that you have been overproducing insulin, which promotes the formation of fat. There's a good chance that, if you are seriously overweight, you also have high blood pressure and/or high cholesterol and triglycerides. Don't get discouraged, though: Remember that you can reverse all of these conditions.

Diet Recommendations

Follow the Anti-X Extra-Healing Diet Plan until four weeks *after* you reach your desired weight. Then slowly shift to the Basic Anti-X Diet Plan, initially by adding some carbohydrates in the form of fruit. If you regain weight quickly, return to the Anti-X Extra-Healing Diet Plan.

Physical Activity

It's sometimes hard to get motivated about any kind of physical activity when you are considerably overweight. So, give yourself a break and focus on only diet and supplements for the first few weeks. Then, after you have shed a few pounds, begin increasing your physical activity, with short walks and walking down stairs at first. As time goes on, strive for longer walks and maybe swimming or even working up a sweat on the dance floor.

Recommended Daily Supplements

Combined with a low-carbohydrate diet and physical activity, some supplements can greatly improve how the body uses insulin and burns glucose—in effect, disposing of carbohydrate calories.

- A high-potency multivitamin supplement
- A multimineral supplement without iron or copper
- Alpha lipoic acid, 50–200 mg
- Chromium, so you are taking a total of 400–800 mcg
- Coenzyme Q_{10} (which helps burn glucose), 50 mg
- Carnitine (which helps transport fats to where they are burned in cells), 500 mg

YOU HAVE HIGH CHOLESTEROL OR HIGH TRIGLYCERIDES . . .

High total cholesterol, low HDL (good) cholesterol, and high triglycerides are risk factors for coronary heart (artery) disease. Keep in mind that dietary cholesterol has relatively little effect on blood levels of this essential fat. Rather, dietary carbohydrates tend to boost both cholesterol and triglyceride levels. In addition, oxidized (free-radical damaged) cholesterol may be more serious than elevated cholesterol per se.

Diet Recommendations

Follow the Anti-X Extra-Healing Diet Plan until your condition improves. Use liberal amounts of garlic and olive oil in your foods. In addition, add avocadoes to your diet; studies have shown them to lower cholesterol levels. Also, try drinking two cups of green tea daily; if you need to, sweeten it with stevia.

You also might try modifying the Anti-X Extra-Healing Diet Plan by adding small portion-controlled servings of oatmeal (½ cup) or half an apple a few times a week; these foods contain a type of fiber that helps lower cholesterol levels.

Physical Activity

Physical activity can lower cholesterol levels, so increase your activity throughout the day. A few ideas: Play catch with your kids, do more yardwork or housework, and take regular walks in the morning, during lunch, or after work.

Recommended Daily Supplements

The following supplements can have a pronounced cholesterol-lowering effect. Consider taking one or more of them, in addition to a multivitamin/mineral supplement without iron or copper.

- Natural beta-carotene from *D. salina* algae, 10 mg
- Fenugreek extract, 5–10 mg daily
- Omega-3 fish oils, 1–3 grams
- Garlic capsules, 800–7,000 mg
- To prevent cholesterol oxidation—400 IU of vitamin E and 1,000 mg of vitamin C

YOU HAVE BEEN DIAGNOSED WITH SYNDROME X . . .

Consider a diagnosis of Syndrome X (the combination of insulin resistance with high cholesterol and triglyceride, hypertension, and/or obesity) as an opportunity to correct long-term dietary and lifestyle problems before they lead to diabetes, heart disease, or other disorders.

Diet Recommendations

Follow the Anti-X Extra-Healing Diet Plan for several months, then graduate to the Basic Anti-X Diet Plan. Sprinkle cinnamon on foods and in drinks, use garlic and onions liberally, and try drinking green tea instead of coffee. Another food-therapy idea to try is to buy unripe bitter melon at an Asian grocery store, and fry it as a side dish a couple times a week.

Physical Activity

The more active you are, the better, but just get started doing something. Gardening gets you out in the sun and helps your body make its own vitamin D, which lowers the risk of Syndrome X. To avoid boredom, vary your activities, though: Go for walks, short bicycle rides, or out dancing.

Recommended Daily Supplements

- Start with AlphaBetic, a once-daily vitamin-mineral supplement.
- Add natural vitamin E, so your intake is in the range of 400–600 IU.
- Add extra vitamin C, so your total intake is 500–1,000 mg.
- Add 300–400 mg of alpha lipoic acid.
- Also take silymarin, 300–400 mg.

YOU HAVE BEEN DIAGNOSED WITH ADULT-ONSET DIABETES . . .

If you have adult-onset (non-insulin-dependent) diabetes, you also have insulin resistance and, probably, at least some of the other characteristic symptoms of Syndrome X. Reversing diabetes is completely within your grasp. The payoff is that you will add healthy years to your life.

Diet Recommendations

Follow the Anti-X Extra-Healing Diet Plan for several months, until your glucose and insulin function, weight, and other symptoms start to normalize. At that point, shift to the Basic Anti-X Diet Plan, and see whether you can continue making progress in reversing your diabetic symptoms. Add small amounts of cinnamon, cloves, and bay leaves to meals—these culinary herbs can improve insulin function. Coriander, another tasty herb, can lower glucose levels.

Physical Activity

Physical activity can accelerate the reversal of diabetic symptoms because it promotes more efficient insulin function and glucose burning. Don't overdo at first—enjoy some walks and swimming. Build up your endurance so, after a few months, you can walk for concentrated periods of time.

Recommended Daily Supplements

- Build your supplement program around AlphaBetic, a once-daily vitamin-mineral supplement designed for diabetics.
- Add extra alpha lipoic acid, so that your total intake is 400–600 mg. (If you are taking medications to lower glucose, you may have to reduce their dosage—work with your physician on this.)
- Add natural vitamin E, so your intake is in the range of 400–600 IU.
- Bring your total vitamin C intake up to 500–1,000 mg.
- Bring your total chromium intake up to 400–1,000 mcg.
- Bring your total zinc intake up to 30–50 mg.
- Bring your magnesium intake up to 400–600 mg.
- Add 140–420 mg of silymarin (or a milk-thistle complex).

YOU HAVE BEEN DIAGNOSED WITH CORONARY HEART DISEASE . . .

Coronary heart disease is caused by more than an accumulation of cholesterol in artery walls. It's the end stage of eating the wrong diet and living the wrong lifestyle for decades. If you've been given the diagnosis of heart disease, see it as an opportunity to make things right. While you probably won't be able to completely reverse years of damage, you can certainly lessen it and give yourself a new lease on life.

Diet Recommendations

Follow the Basic Anti-X Diet Plan or, if your condition is severe, the Anti-X Extra-Healing Diet Plan. Try to use plenty of garlic and onions in your cooking, and eat cold-water fish several times a week.

Physical Activity

Lack of physical activity is comparable to smoking as a risk factor for coronary heart disease. To reduce this risk, you've got to begin somewhere, so start with daily walks or an occasional light swim. Be careful not to push yourself too hard at first. Start slowly, and build up your endurance.

Recommended Daily Supplements

- Take a high-potency multivitamin.
- Take a multimineral supplement without iron or copper.
- Add natural vitamin E, so your total intake is 400–800 IU.
- Add vitamin C, so your total intake is 1,000 mg.
- Add coenzyme Q_{10}, 100 mg.
- Add alpha lipoic acid, 100 mg.
- Optional: Take Pycnogenol, 50 mg.

Finally, if you are taking medications or are seriously ill, recognize that you may benefit greatly from the guidance of a nutritionally oriented physician. Such a physician may recommend higher dosages of some of these supplements, but she or he also has the advantage of monitoring your progress as a patient. To get a referral to a nutritionally oriented doctor, enter your zip code in the website for the American College for Advancement in Medicine (ACAM): www.acam.org.

Some Final Words

THE STORY OF SYNDROME X reads somewhat like a mystery novel in which a detective must study the clues (some of which may not be entirely obvious), figure out how to connect the pieces of evidence, identify the true culprit, and solve the problem.

Some of the clues to our modern maladies are insulin resistance, obesity, high blood pressure, and elevated levels of cholesterol and triglycerides. Most people—indeed, most physicians—have failed to connect them. They see these disorders as unrelated risk factors for heart disease and diabetes. However, the truth of the matter is that these disorders *are* related to each other. Together, they constitute Syndrome X, and they significantly increase the risk of heart disease, diabetes, and other age-related degenerative diseases.

By connecting the pieces of this story, it becomes clear that the culprit in this mystery is not so much genetics or cruel fate, but a modern diet built around abnormally large quantities of sugars and other refined carbohydrates. Eating these foods causes rapid rises in glucose and insulin, as well as nutrient deficiencies, all of which lead to Syndrome X and associated disorders.

By connecting a few more pieces, you discover that Syndrome X and its characteristic symptoms *are* preventable and reversible. The key to solving this mystery is remembering that human beings evolved eating diets high in animal protein, vegetables, vitamins, and minerals, and low in refined sugars and other carbohydrates. This is the type of diet that protects against Syndrome X.

Like any good detective, once you've solved the mystery behind your health problems, it's time to put your knowledge into action. To protect yourself against Syndrome X, you need to "go against the grain"—figuratively and literally—and make a conscious effort to carefully select foods that keep you healthy. These foods are high in protein, contain a balance of dietary fats, and provide only the most natural carbohydrates, such as those found in nonstarchy vegetables.

Eating this way may initially take a little getting used to, but there are plenty of payoffs for this dietary discipline. You will, of course, feel better very quickly, and over the long term, you will reduce your risk of developing disease. You'll probably also look better, trimmer, and younger than those who don't have the Anti-X advantage. If you're like most people, you will also find the Anti-X diet easy to follow and far tastier than the diet you've been eating. It usually doesn't take long before this way of eating feels completely natural—because it makes you feel *so good*.

As you begin, remember that your health is the most precious possession you have. With it, you have the opportunity to accomplish everything else you want in life. Without your health, everything you desire will start to slip through your fingers. What we have written in this book gives you the guidance to maintain and, if necessary, restore your health. Use it and live life to its fullest.

APPENDIX A

Resources

There are many important resources you can use in educating yourself further on nutrition and health, supplements, and preventing and reversing Syndrome X. Here are some of them.

MAGAZINES AND NEWSLETTERS

The Nutrition Reporter

This monthly newsletter summarizes recent research on vitamins, minerals, and herbs. The annual subscription rate is $25 ($48 CND for Canada, $38 U.S. funds for all other countries). For a sample issue, send a business-size self-addressed stamped envelope (SASE), with postage for two ounces, to *The Nutrition Reporter*, Post Office Box 30246, Tucson, AZ 85751-0246.

Let's Live Magazine

This monthly magazine focuses on how diet, nutrition, and supplements help maintain health and reverse disease. The annual subscription is $15.95. To order, call 1-800-365-3790.

Natural Health Magazine

Natural Health eclectically covers the entire range of natural health—supplements, herbs, home remedies, diet, food, and lifestyle. Its articles are well researched and thorough. The annual subscription is $17.95. 1-800-526-8440.

Country Living's Healthy Living Magazine

This spinoff of *Country Living* is well written and lively. It covers supplements, fitness, diet, and recipes. The annual subscription is $15. 1-800-925-0485.

Great Life

This monthly magazine, purchased by many health-food retailers throughout the country, is distributed to consumers free of charge. Its articles focus on the use of supplements and diet to promote health and are written primarily by science, medical, and health professionals.

Delicious!

Another complimentary publication distributed by natural-food stores, *Delicious!* began as a food magazine for the natural-foods industry, but it now covers a wide array of natural health topics. Especially noteworthy are its recipes, which show how to combine vegetables in tasty, innovative ways. For information on individual subscriptions, call 303-998-9390, or visit the magazine online at www.healthwell.com.

SUGGESTED HEALTH BOOKS TO READ

There are many excellent books that provide additional information about the roles of nutrition and supplements in health. These are some of them.

Books about Food and Diet

The Anti-Aging Zone, by Barry Sears, Ph.D. (ReganBooks, 1999, $25.00). An in-depth, technical look at how a balanced diet, moderate in carbohydrates, slows the aging process.

Get the Sugar Out, by Ann Louise Gittleman, M.S., C.N.S. (Crown Trade Paper-backs, 1996, $11.00). An easy-to-read book offering 501 consumer-friendly sugges-tions on how to reduce sugar intake; it also has more than 50 low-sugar, naturally sweetened recipes, including low-sugar versions of pumpkin pie, birthday cake, pudding, and other desserts.

The High Blood Pressure Solution: Natural Prevention and Cure with the K Factor, by Richard D. Moore, M.D., Ph.D. (Healing Arts Press, 1993, $12.95). A detailed explanation of how a diet rich in potassium and low in sodium helps prevent and treat hypertension.

The Omega Plan, by Artemis P. Simopoulos, M.D., and Jo Robinson (HarperCollins, 1998, $24.00). A consumer-friendly book that explains how lowering the intake of omega-6 fatty acids in the diet and increasing omega-3 fats and monounsaturated fats can reduce not only the risk of insulin resistance, overweight, and Syndrome X, but also the risk of a wide range of other conditions, including cancer, depres-sion, and autoimmune diseases.

The Paleolithic Prescription, by S. Boyd Eaton, M.D., Marjorie Shostak, and Melvin Konner, M.D, Ph.D. (Harper & Row, 1989, $8.95). The classic book on the diet that the human race evolved on, by the true experts on this topic; unfortunately, now out of print, but may be available in libraries and used bookstores.

Protein Power, by Michael R. Eades, M.D., and Mary Dan Eades, M.D. (Bantam Books, 1996, $21.95). A good explanation of how high-carbohydrate diets lead to insulin resistance and Syndrome X and how changing the diet can correct these conditions.

The Stevia Cookbook, by Ray Sahelian, M.D., and Donna Gates (Avery Publishing, 1999, $12.95). Explains the little-known history and benefits of the herb stevia and tells how to replace sugar with stevia in recipes. Contains more than 100 no-sugar recipes for everything from French salad dressing to chocolate truffles.

Books about Nutritional Supplements

The Alpha Lipoic Acid Breakthrough, by Burt Berkson, M.D. (Prima Publishing, 1998, $12.95). *The* book on alpha lipoic acid for consumers, covering its use in diabetes, mushroom poisoning, nerve disorders, and aging.

The Antioxidant Miracle, by Lester Packer, Ph.D., and Carol Colman (John Wiley & Sons, 1999, $24.95). In reader-friendly terms, explains the *antioxidant network—* the combination of antioxidants that work together, synergistically, to fight off disease and aging.

The Avery FAQs series, consisting of several dozen paperback books with information on nutrition, supplements, and disease prevention in an easy-to-read question-and-answer format; some titles include *All about Zinc, All about Vitamin E, All about Chromium Picolinate,* and *All about Diabetes.* (Avery Publishing Group, 1998–2000, $2.99 each, 1-800-548-5757).

Dr. Atkins' Vita-Nutrient Solution, by Robert C. Atkins, M.D. (Simon & Schuster, 1998, $24.00). An easy-to-read yet comprehensive reference book that provides information and dosage recommendations on a wide range of supplements, including vitamins, minerals, amino acids, fats, digestive aids, and herbs.

Encyclopedia of Nutritional Supplements, by Michael T. Murray, N.D. (Prima Publishing, 1996, $19.95). Another comprehensive, well-referenced guide to vitamins, minerals, essential fatty acids, accessory nutrients, and glandular products.

The Green Pharmacy, by James A. Duke, Ph.D. (St. Martin Paperbacks, 1997, $6.99). The ultimate, user-friendly guide to herbal remedies by one of the top experts in the country.

Books about Other Topics of Interest

Healthy Pleasures, by Robert Ornstein, Ph.D., and David Sobel, M.D. (Addison-Wesley Publishing, 1989, $6.95). Introduces the reader to the scientifically proven health benefits of pleasure; contains an excellent chapter on physical activity entitled, "Why Kill Yourself to Save Your Life?"

Walking: A Complete Guide to the Complete Exercise, by Casey Meyers (Random House, 1992, $12.00). A comprehensive book that explains why walking is a better exercise than running and how you can embark on a walking program for life to keep you in tip-top shape.

COMPANIES THAT PRODUCE AND SELL NATURAL-FOOD PRODUCTS

Health- and natural-food stores really matured during the 1990s. Many cities have several Whole Foods and Wild Oats natural supermarkets, as well as independently owned stores.

Allergy Resources
1-719-488-3630
1-800-USE-FLAX
A mail-order company that sells a wide selection of natural and alternative food and health products, including hard-to-find food items mentioned in this book, such as flaxseed oil and stevia.

Body Ecology
1-800-511-2660 (USA)
1-800-896-7838 (Canada)
www.bodyecology.net
The Body Ecology Company is a source for stevia and for books with sugar-free recipes that use stevia.

Born 3 Marketing Company
1-604-856-1243
A Canadian source of omega-3 fortified eggs.

The Country Hen
1-508-928-5333
A producer of omega-3-enriched eggs sold throughout the northeast section of the United States. Each egg contains 170 mg of omega-3 fatty acids.

ERBL, Inc.
1-760-599-6088
Makers of an innovative source of omega-3 fish oils, Coromega—a natural-orange flavor, sugar-free, pudding-like mixture. It's especially great for kids who won't eat fish.

French Meadow Bakery
1-612-870-4740
French Meadow Bakery produces tasty whole-grain sourdough breads made with unrefined sea salt instead of commercial table salt, including spelt sourdough, which contains 10 grams of carbohydrates per slice, and rye-linseed that has omega-3-rich flaxseeds.

Gold Circle Farms
1-888-599-4DHA
www.goldcirclefarms.com

Gold Circle Farms produces eggs that are naturally enriched with beneficial omega-3 fatty acids and vitamin E. They're becoming increasingly available in regular commercial supermarkets, especially in the western United States. Each egg contains 175 mg omega-3 fats and 6 IU vitamin E.

Mental Processes
1-800-431-4018
www.pumpkorn.com
Mental Processes is the manufacturer of Pumpkorn, a tasty, healthy snack food made out of pumpkin seeds—seeds that contain a good balance of healthy fats and protein and are high in zinc. Pumpkorn comes in several varieties, including original, chili-flavored, curry, and maple-vanilla.

Northwest Natural
1-360-866-9661
This small but quality-minded company markets frozen fish products that are convenient sources of beneficial omega-3 fatty acids. Northwest Natural makes three products: salmon burgers, halibut burgers, and tuna with pesto medallions, which are available at natural-food stores throughout the United States.

Omega Nutrition
1-800-661-3529
www.omegaflo.com
Omega Nutrition is arguably the producer of the best vegetable oils on the market; the oils are unrefined, organic, and minimally processed. In addition to selling high-quality oils (which can be shipped directly to your home), the company also is a one-stop shop for other helpful products, such as stevia and informative books on stevia, healthy fats, and other nutrition topics of interest.

Organic Food Products, Inc.
1-408-782-1133
Organic Food Products is the producer of Millina's Healthy Kitchen pasta sauces, which come in three tasty varieties: marinara, tomato garlic, and tomato basil. These sauces contain organic ingredients, have no added sugar, and are enriched with omega-3 fatty acids (without a fishy taste).

Pilgrim's Pride EggsPlus
1-800-824-1159
Pilgrim's Pride, the fifth largest poultry company in the United States, is now offering omega-3-fortified eggs to the national market. Each egg contains 200 mg omega-3 fatty acids.

Whole Foods
www.wholefoods.com
With stores in 21 states, Whole Foods is the largest nationwide chain of natural-food stores. The emphasis is on wholesome, natural foods, including fresh organically produced meats, organic produce, and a wide variety of other healthful food products.

Wild Oats
1-800-494-WILD
www.wildoats.com
This nationwide chain of natural-food stores operates in 18 states and British Columbia (Canada). Unlike the health-food stores of the past, Wild Oats stores are as consumer-friendly as the best supermarkets. The emphasis is on natural and gourmet food products, with organically grown produce and organically produced meat and groceries.

Zeus Mediterranean Foods
1-843-207-1040
www.zeusfoods.com
Zeus Foods is the producer of a line of authentic Greek salad dressings. The products can be found in an increasing number of supermarkets and gourmet food stores across the country. The dressings are made with extra-virgin olive oil and canola oil and are free of added sugar and/or preservatives.

COMPANIES THAT SELL VITAMINS, MINERALS, AND HERBAL SUPPLEMENTS

In general, we recommend that you purchase supplements from companies that have historically sold their products in health-food stores. Such brands are generally manufactured without sugar, artificial colorings, and common allergy-provoking ingredients.

Abkit/NatureWorks
1-800-226-6227
Abkit manufactures and markets AlphaBetic, a once-daily multivitamin/multimineral supplement designed for diabetics. Unlike nearly all other supplements of this sort, it contains alpha lipoic acid and chromium. Although the dosages are modest, it is an excellent supplement for people with Syndrome X or diabetes. Abkit also manufactures and markets Alpha-Lipotene, an excellent alpha lipoic acid supplement, under its NatureWorks label.

Advanced Physicians Products (APP)
1-800-220-7687
(Ask for the catalog with Syndrome X–related products.)
http://www.nutritiononline.com
Founded by a nutritionally oriented physician, APP offers a broad line of excellent vitamin and mineral products, many of which are helpful to people with Syndrome X. Among the products are alpha lipoic acid (by itself and as part of a multivitamin), natural vitamin E, mixed carotenoids, and vitamin C.

Alacer
1-800-854-0249
http://www.alacercorp.com
Alacer manufactures some of the most distinctive vitamin C products in the marketplace. Most are tasty 1-gram packets of vitamin C, with minerals, which can be

mixed in a glass of water. Most of the vitamin C products are sweetened with fructose, though, so avoid these and opt for the company's unsweetened (but tasty) "Lite" ones instead.

Bioforce
1-877-232-6060
www.bioforce.com
Bioforce is a venerable Swiss maker of herbal products—mostly tinctures, but also some tablets and ointments. The company's milk-thistle complex is an excellent product. The products are not standardized in the conventional sense, but the company's manufacturing controls ensure exceptional consistency and quality.

Eclectic Institute
1-800-332-4372
The Eclectic Institute, which is a supplement company and not an "institute," sells a number of freeze-dried and liquid-extract herbal supplements. Some of the supplements, such as bitter melon, are very difficult to find elsewhere in supplemental form.

J. R. Carlson Laboratories
1-800-323-4141
www.carlsonlabs.com
Carlson Labs is the premier maker and distributor of a wide range of natural vitamin E products, including supplements, creams, ointments, suppositories, and more. The company sells a wide range of other vitamin and mineral supplements, as well.

L & H Vitamins
1-800-221-1152
This mail-order company sells many leading health-food brands of supplements at discounted prices.

Nature's Way
1-801-489-1500
www.naturesway.com
Nature's Way is a leading herb-supplement company, with most of its 350 products sold in capsule form. Some of the company's products are standardized; others are whole-herb products.

Nutricology/Allergy Research Group
1-800-545-9960
www.nutricology.com
Nutricology/Allergy Research Group is one of the most innovative companies in terms of developing useful supplements.

Thorne Research
1-208-263-1337
www.thorne.com
Thorne is one of the most ethical supplement companies we've found, and its product quality is exceptionally high. The company's principal customers are physicians, but it won't turn away a consumer order. It produces multimineral supplements, such as Biomins II, without iron and copper.

Vitaline
1-800-648-4755
www.vitaline.com
This company is best known for its coenzyme Q_{10} products, which have been shown to be clinically effective. Vitaline also sells a growing line of other vitamin and mineral supplements.

Vitamin Shoppe
1-800-223-1216
This mail-order company sells most leading health-food brands of supplements, discounted by 25–30 percent, which can lead to a hefty savings.

WEBSITES

http://www.nutritionreporter.com
For articles on research related to the use of nutrition and dietary supplements.

http://www.syndrome-x.com
For information on Syndrome X.

TESTING LABORATORIES

Most testing laboratories prefer to work with physicians. These three laboratories are set up to analyze nutrient levels. Physicians and local clinical laboratories can prepare blood for shipment to them.

Bright Spot for Health
1-316-682-3100
www.brightspot.org

Great Smokies Diagnostic Laboratory
1-800-522-4762
www.greatsmokies-lab.com

Pantox Laboratories
1-619-272-3885
www.pantox.com

APPENDIX B

Selected References

Chapter 1. The Food-Health Connection

Bogert LJ, *Nutrition and Physical Fitness*, Philadelphia: Saunders, 1939:437

Opara IU, Levine JH, "The deadly quartet—the insulin resistance syndrome," *Southern Medical Journal*, 1997;90:1162–1168.

Pyorala M, Miettinen H, Laakso M, et al., "Hyperinsulinemia predicts coronary heart disease risk in healthy middle-age men: The 22-year follow-up results of the Helsinki policeman study," *Circulation*, 1998;98:398–404.

Reaven GM, "Pathophysiology of insulin resistance in human disease," *Physiological Reviews*, 1995; 75:473–485.

Williams KV, Korytkowski MT, "Syndrome X: Pathogenesis, clinical and therapeutic aspects," *Diabetes Nutrition and Metabolism*, 1998;11:140–152.

Chapter 2. Understanding Glucose and Insulin

Boden G, Chen X, Ruiz J, "Mechanisms of fatty acid-induced inhibition of glucose uptake," *Journal of Clinical Investigation*, 1994;93:2438–2446.

Chen Y-D, Coulston AM, Zhou M-Y, et al., "Why do low-fat high-carbohydrate diets accentuate postprandial lipemia in patients with NIDDM?" *Diabetes Care*, 1995;18:10–16.

Torjeson PA, Birkeland KI, Anderssen SA, et al., "Lifestyle changes may reverse development of the insulin resistance syndrome," *Diabetes Care*, 1997;20:26–31.

Wells AS, Read NW, Laugharne JDF, et al., "Alterations in mood after changing to a low-fat diet," *British Journal of Nutrition*, 1998;79.23–30.

Chapter 3. Syndrome X: Unconnected Symptoms, Connected Causes

Carantoni M, Abbasi F, Warmerdam F, et al., "Relationship between insulin resistance and partially oxidized LDL particles in healthy, nondiabetic volunteers," *Arteriosclerosis, Thrombosis and Vascular Biology*, 1998;18:762–767.

Facchini FS, Stoohs RA, Reaven GM, "Enhanced sympathetic nervous system activity: The linchpin between insulin resistance, hyperinsulinemia, and heart rate," *American Journal of Hypertension*, 1996;9:1013–1017.

Gaziano JM, Hennekens CH, O'Donnel CJ, et al., "Fasting triglycerides, high-density lipoprotein, and risk of myocardial infarction," *Circulation*, 1997;96: 2520–2525.

Maheux P, Jeppesen J, Sheu WH, et al., "Additive effects of obesity, hypertension and type 2 diabetes on insulin resistance," *Hypertension*, 1994;24:695–698.

Mau MK, Grandinetti A, Arakaki R, "The insulin resistance syndrome in native Hawaiians," *Diabetes Care*, 1997;20:1376–1380.

Plotnick GD, Corretti MC, Vogel RA, "Effect of antioxidant vitamins on the transient impairment of endothelium-dependent brachial artery vasoactivity following a single high-fat meal," *JAMA*, 1997;278:1682–1686.

Reaven GM, "Role of insulin resistance in human disease," *Diabetes*, 1988;37:1595–1607.

Trevisan M, Liu J, Hahsas FB, et al., "Syndrome X and mortality: A population-based study," *American Journal of Epidemiology*, 1998;148:958–966.

Chapter 4. Beyond Syndrome X: Sugar and Insulin Overload

Ceriello A, Bortolotti N, Crescentini A, et al., "Antioxidant defences are reduced during the oral glucose tolerance test in normal and noninsulin-dependent diabetic subjects," *European Journal of Clinical Investigation*, 1998;28:329–333.

Ceriello A, Bortolotti N, Motz E, et al., "Meal-generated oxidative stress in type 2 diabetic patients," *Diabetes Care*, 1998;21:1529–1533.

Ceriello A, Bortolotti N, Pirisi M, et al., "Total plasma antioxidant capacity predicts thrombosis-prone status in NIDDM patients," *Diabetes Care*, 1997;20:1589–1593.

Cleland SJ, Petrie JR, Ueda S, et al., "Insulin as a vascular hormone: Implications for the pathophysiology of cardiovascular disease," *Clinical and Experimental Pharmacology and Physiology*, 1998;25:175–184.

De Stefani E, Deneo-Pellegrini H, Mendilaharsu M, et al., "Dietary sugar and lung cancer: A case-control study in Uruguay," *Nutrition and Cancer*, 1998;31:132–137.

Ely JTA, "Glycemic modulation of tumor tolerance," *Journal of Orthomolecular Medicine*, 1996;11: 23–34.

Faure P, Rossini E, Lafond JL, "Vitamin E improves the free radical defense system potential and insulin sensitivity of rats fed high fructose diets," *Journal of Nutrition*, 1997;127:103–107.

Jeppeson J, Chen Y-DI, Zhou M-Y, "Postprandial triglyceride and retinyl ester responses to oral fat: Effects of fructose," *American Journal of Clinical Nutrition*, 1995;61:781–791.

Keltikangas-Jarvinen L, Raikkonen K, Hautanen A, et al., "Vital exhaustion, anger expression, and pituitary and adrenocorticol hormones," *Arteriosclerosis, Thrombosis and Vascular Biology*, 1996; 16:275–280.

Kijak E, Foust G, Steinman RR, "Relationship of blood sugar level and leukocyte phagocytosis," *Journal of the Southern California Dental Association*, 1964;32:349–351.

Koohestani N, Tran TT, Lee W, et al., "Insulin resistance and promotion of aberrant crypt foci in the colons of rats on a high-fat diet," *Nutrition and Cancer*, 1997;29:69–76.

Kunisaki M, Umeda F, Inoguchi T, "Effects of vitamin E administration on platelet function in diabetes mellitus," *Diabetes Research*, 1990;14:37–42.

La Vecchia C, Negri E, Franceschi S, et al., "A case-control study of diabetes mellitus and cancer risk," *British Journal of Cancer*, 1994;70:950–953.

Lamarche B, Tchernof A, Mauriege P, et al., "Fasting insulin and apolipoprotein B levels and low-density lipoprotein particle size as risk factors for ischemic heart disease," *JAMA*, 1998;279: 1955–1961.

Lee BM, Wolever TMS, "Effect of glucose, sucrose and fructose on plasma glucose and insulin responses in normal humans: Comparison with white bread," *European Journal of Clinical Nutrition*, 1998;52:924–928.

Levi B, Werman MJ, "Long-term fructose consumption accelerates glycation and several age-related variables in male rats," *Journal of Nutrition*, 1998;128:1442–1449.

Lev-Ran A, "Mitogenic factors accelerate later-age diseases: Insulin as a paradigm," *Mechanisms of Aging and Development*, 1998;102:95–113.

Liu S, Stampfer JM, Manson JE, et al., "A prospective study of dietary glycemic load and risk of myocardial infarction in women," presented at Experimental Biology 98, San Francisco, California, April 18–22, 1998.

Masoro EJ, Katz MS, McMahan CA, "Evidence for the glycation hypothesis of aging from the food-restricted rodent model," *Journal of Gerontology*, 1989;44:820–822.

Maxwell SRJ, Thomason H, Sandler D, "Antioxidant status in patients with uncomplicated insulin-dependent and non-insulin-dependent diabetes mellitus," *European Journal of Clinical Investigation*, 1997;27:484–490.

Nielsen FH, Milne DB, "Dietary fructose and magnesium affect macromineral metabolism in men," *Proceedings of the North Dakota Academy of Science*, 1997;51:212.

Nourooz-Zadeh J, Rahimi A, Tajaddini-Sarmadi J, et al., "Relationships between plasma measures of oxidative stress and metabolic control in NIDDM," *Diabetologia*, 1997;40:647–653.

Sanchez JL, et al., "Role of sugars in human neutrophilic phagocytosis," *American Journal of Clinical Nutrition*, 1973;26:1180–1184.

Sharpe PC, Yue KKM, Catherwood MA, et al., "The effects of glucose-induced oxidative stress on growth and extracellular matrix gene expression of vascular smooth muscle cells," *Diabetologia*, 1998;41:1210–1219.

Chapter 5. The Case for Nutritional Therapies over Drugs

Bendich A, Mallick R, Leader S, "Potential health economic benefits of vitamin supplementation," *Western Journal of Medicine*, 1997;166:306–312.

Carlsen SM, Folling I, Grill V, et al., "Metformin increases total serum homocysteine levels in non-diabetic male patients with coronary heart disease," *Scandinavian Journal of Clinical and Laboratory Investigation,* 1997;57:521–527.

de Lorgeril M, Salen P, Martin J-L, et al., "Mediterranean diet, traditional risk factors, and the rate of cardiovascular complications after myocardial infarction," *Circulation,* 1999;99:779–785.

Hoffman C, Rice D, Sung H-Y, "Persons with chronic conditions: Their prevalence and costs," *JAMA,* 1996;276:1473–1479.

Lazarou J, Pomeranz BH, Corey PN, "Incidence of adverse drug reactions in hospitalized patients: A meta-analysis of prospective studies," *JAMA,* 1998;279:1200–1205.

Phillips DP, Christenfield N, Glynn LM, "Increase in US medication-error deaths between 1983 and 1993," *Lancet,* 1998;351:643–644.

Chapter 6. The Diet We Were Made For and How It Changed

Eaton SB, Eaton SB III, Konner MJ, et al., "An evolutionary perspective enhances understanding of human nutritional requirements," *Journal of Nutrition,* 1996;126:1732–1740.

Eaton SB, Eaton SB III, Konner MJ, "Paleolithic nutrition revisited: A twelve-year retrospective on its nature and implications," *European Journal of Clinical Nutrition,* 1997;51:207–216.

Eaton SB, Shostak M, Konner M, *The Paleolithic Prescription,* New York: Harper and Row, 1988:78.

Chapter 7. Redefining What to Eat: The Nine Anti-X Diet Principles

Ascherio A, Willett WC, "Health effects of trans fatty acids," *American Journal of Clinical Nutrition,* 1997;66(suppl):1006S–1010S.

Axelrod L, Kleinman K, et al., "Effects of a small quantity of omega-3 fatty acids on cardiovascular risk factors in NIDDM," *Diabetes Care,* 1994;17:37–44.

Fanaian M, Szilasi J, Storlien L, et al., "The effect of modified fat diet on insulin resistance and metabolic parameters in type II diabetes," *Diabetologia,* 1996;39:A7.

Garg A, "High-monounsaturated-fat diets for patients with diabetes mellitus: A meta-analysis," *American Journal of Clinical Nutrition,* 1998;67(suppl):577S–582S.

Kuller LH (letter), *Lancet,* 1993;341:1093–1094.

Moore RD, *The High Blood Pressure Solution: Natural Prevention and Cure with the K Factor,* Rochester, Vt.: Healing Arts Press, 1993.

Salmeron J, Manson JE, Stampfer MJ, et al., "Dietary fiber, glycemic load, and the risk of non-insulin-dependent diabetes mellitus in women," *JAMA,* 1997;277:472–477.

Storlien LH, "Skeletal muscle membrane lipids and insulin resistance," *Lipids,* 1996;31(suppl): S261–265.

Torjesen PA, et al., "Lifestyle changes may reverse development of the insulin resistance syndrome," *Diabetes Care,* 1997;30:26–31.

Chapter 10. A Rational Approach to Fitness and Physical Activity

Anderson RE, Wadden TA, Bartlett SJ, et al., "Effects of lifestyle activity vs. structured aerobic exercise in obese women," *JAMA,* 1999;281:335–340.

Dunn AL, Marcus BH, Kampert JB, et al., "Comparison of lifestyle and structured interventions to increase physical activity and cardiorespiratory fitness," *JAMA,* 1999;281:327–334.

Helmrich SP, Ragland DR, Leung RW, et al., "Physical activity and reduced occurrence of non-insulin-dependent diabetes mellitus," *New England Journal of Medicine,* 1991;325:147–152.

Mayer-Davis EJ, D'Agostino R, Karter AJ, et al., "Intensity and amount of physical activity in relation to insulin sensitivity," *JAMA,* 1998;279:669–674.

Chapter 11. Alpha Lipoic Acid: The Master Nutrient

Cameron NE, Cotter MA, Horrobin DH, et al., "Effects of α-lipoic acid on neurovascular function in diabetic rats: Interaction with essential fatty acids," *Diabetologia,* 1998;41:390–399.

Jacob S, Henriksen EJ, Ruus P, et al., "The radical scavenger α-lipoic acid enhances insulin sensitivity in patients with NIDDM: A placebo-controlled trial," presented at Oxidants and Antioxidants in Biology, Santa Barbara, Calif., February 26–March 1, 1997.

Jacob S, Henriksen EJ, Schiemann AL, et al., "Enhancement of glucose disposal in patients with type 2 diabetes by alpha-lipoic acid," *Arzneimittel-Forschung Drug Research,* 1995;45:872–874.

Jacob S, Streeper RS, Fogt DL, et al., "The antioxidant α-lipoic acid enhances insulin-stimulated glucose metabolism in insulin-resistant rat skeletal muscle," *Diabetes,* 1996;45:1024–1029.

Jain SK, Lim G, "Lipoic acid (LA) decreases protein glycation and increases (Na++K+)- and Ca++-ATPases activities in high glucose (G)-treated red blood cells (RBC)," *Free Radical Biology and Medicine*, 1998;25:S94, Abstract #268.

Khamaisi M, Potashnik R, Tirosh A, et al., "Lipoic acid reduces glycemia and increases muscle GLUT4 content in streptozotocin-diabetic rats," *Metabolism*, 1997;46:763–768.

Konrad T, Vivina P, Kusterer K, et al., "α-lipoic acid treatment decreases serum lactate and pyruvate concentrations and improves glucose effectiveness in lean and obese patients with type 2 diabetes," *Diabetes Care*, 1999;22:280–287.

Rett K, Wicklmayr M, Ruus P, et al., "Alpha-liponsäure (Thioactsäure) steigert die Insulinempfindlichkeit übergewichtiger Patienten mit Type-II-Diabetes," *Diabetes und Stoffwechsel*, 1996; 5(suppl 3):59–62.

Chapter 12. Vitamin E: The Cardiovascular Nutrient

Heinonen OP, Albanes D, Virtano J, et al., "Prostate cancer and supplementation with α-tocopherol and β-carotene: Incidence and mortality in a controlled trial," *Journal of the National Cancer Institute*, 1998;90:440–446.

Hodis HN, Mack WJ, BaBree L, et al., "Serial coronary angiographic evidence that antioxidant vitamin intake reduces progression of coronary artery atherosclerosis," *JAMA*, 1995;273:1849–1854.

Ishii K, Zhen LX, Wang DH, et al., "Prevention of mammary tumorigenesis in acatalasemic mice by vitamin E supplementation," *Japanese Journal of Cancer Research*, 1996;87:680–684.

Meydani SN, Meydani M, Blumberg JB, et al., "Vitamin E supplementation and in vivo immune response in healthy elderly subjects," *JAMA*, 1997;277:1380–1386.

Omer B, Akkose A, Kolanci C, et al., "Inhibition of mammary carcinogenesis in rats by parenteral high-dose vitamin E," *Journal of the National Cancer Institute*, 1997;89:972–973.

Plotnick GD, Corretti MC, Vogel RA, "Effect of antioxidant vitamins on the transient impairment of endothelium-dependent brachial artery vasoreactivity following a single high-fat meal," *JAMA*, 1997;278:1682–1686.

Qureshi AA, Qureshi N, Wright JJ, et al., "Lowering of serum cholesterol in hypercholesterolemic humans by tocotrienols (palmvitee)," *American Journal of Clinical Nutrition*, 1991;53(suppl 4): 1021S–1026S.

Rimm EB, Stampfer MJ, Ascherio A, et al., "Vitamin E consumption and the risk of coronary heart disease in men," *New England Journal of Medicine*, 1993;328:1450–1456.

Sano M, Ernesto C, Thomas RG, et al., "A controlled trial of selegilin, alpha-tocopherol, or both as treatment for Alzheimer's disease," *New England Journal of Medicine*, 1997;336:1216–1222.

Stampfer MJ, Hennekens CH, Manson JE, et al., "Vitamin E consumption and the risk of coronary heart disease in women," *New England Journal of Medicine*, 1993;328:1444–1449.

Chapter 13. Vitamin C: The Well-Being Nutrient

Cameron E, Pauling L, *Cancer and Vitamin C*, Menlo Park, Calif.: Linus Pauling Institute of Science and Medicine, 1979.

Challem JJ, "Views on vitamin C and cancer: An interview with Linus Pauling, Ph.D.," *Let's Live*, January, 1991.

Eriksson J, Kohvakka A, "Magnesium and ascorbic acid supplementation in diabetes mellitus," *Annals of Nutrition and Metabolism*, 1995;39:217–223.

Freyschuss A, Xiu R-J, Zhang J, et al., "Vitamin C reduces cholesterol-induced microcirculatory changes in rabbits," *Arteriosclerosis, Thrombosis, and Vascular Biology*, 1997;17:1178–1184.

Gatto LM, Hallen GK, Brown AJ, et al., "Ascorbic acid induces a favorable lipoprotein profile in women," *Journal of the American College of Nutrition*, 1996;15:154–158.

Hoffer A, Pauling L, "Hardin Jones biostatistical analysis of mortality data for a second set of cohorts of cancer patients with a large fraction surviving at the termination of the study and a comparison of survival times of cancer patients receiving large regular oral doses of vitamin C and other nutrients with similar patients not receiving these doses," *Journal of Orthomolecular Medicine*, 1993;8:157–167.

Johnston CS, Thompson LL, "Vitamin C status of an outpatient population," *Journal of the American College of Nutrition*, 1998;17:366–370.

Johnston CS, Yen M-F, "Megadose of vitamin C delays insulin response to a glucose challenge in normoglycemic adults," *American Journal of Clinical Nutrition*, 1994;60:735–738.

Simon JA, Hudes ES, Browner WS, "Serum ascorbic acid and cardiovascular disease prevalence in U.S. adults," *Epidemiology*, 1998;9:316–321.

Chapter 14. Chromium, Zinc, Magnesium, and Other Minerals

Anderson RA, Chen N, Bryden NA, et al., "Elevated intakes of supplemental chromium improve glucose and insulin variables in individuals with type 2 diabetes," *Diabetes,* 1997;46:1786–1791.

Chen MD, Lin PY, Lin WH, et al., "Zinc in hair and serum of obese individuals," *American Journal of Clinical Nutrition,* 1988;48:1307–1309.

Kaats GR, Blum K, Fisher JA, et al., "Effects of chromium picolinate supplementation on body composition: A randomized, double-masked, placebo-controlled study," *Current Therapeutic Research,* 1996;57:747–756.

Kaats GR, Blum K, Pullin D, et al., "A randomized, double-masked, placebo-controlled study of the effects of chromium picolinate supplementation on body composition: A replication and extension of a previous study," *Current Therapeutic Research,* 1998;59;379–388.

Lee NA, Reasner CA, "Beneficial effect of chromium supplementation on serum triglyceride levels in NIDDM," *Diabetes Care,* 1994;17:1449–1452.

Lukassiak J, Cajzer D, Dabrowska E, et al., "Low zinc levels in metabolic X syndrome (mzX) patients," *Rocz Panstw Zakl Hig,* 1998;49:241–244.

Kao WH, Brancati F, Nieto J, et al., "Serum magnesium concentration and the risk of incident NIDDM: The Atherosclerosis Risk in Communities (ARIC) study," *Diabetes,* 1997;46(Suppl 1)·20A.

Mantzoros CS, Prasad AS, Beck F, et al., "Zinc may regulate serum leptin concentrations in humans," *Journal of the American College of Nutrition* 1998;17:270–275.

Mukherjee B, Anbazhaga S, Roy A, et al., "Novel implications of the potential role of selenium on antioxidant status in streptozotocin-induced diabetic mice," *Biomedicine and Pharmacotherapy,* 1998;52:89–95.

Paolisso G, Sgambato S, Gambardella A, et al., "Daily magnesium supplements improve glucose handling in elderly subjects," *American Journal of Clinical Nutrition,* 1992;55:1161–1167.

Preuss HG, Jarrell ST, Scheckenbach R, et al., "Comparative effects of chromium, vanadium and *Gymnema sylvestre* on sugar-induced blood pressure elevations in SHR," *Journal of the American College of Nutrition,* 1998;17:116–123.

Singh RB, Mohammed AN, Rastogi SS, et al., "Current zinc intake and risk of diabetes and coronary artery disease and factors associated with insulin resistance in rural and urban populations of north India," *Journal of the American College of Nutrition,* 1998;17:564–570.

Verma S, Cam MC, McNeill JH, "Nutritional factors that can favorably influence the glucose/insulin system: Vanadium," *Journal of the American College of Nutrition,* 1998;1·11–18.

Walter RM, Uriu-Hare JY, Olin KS, et al., "Copper, zinc, manganese and magnesium status and complications of diabetes mellitus," *Diabetes Care,* 1991;14:1050–1056.

Chapter 15. A Few More Helpful Nutrients

Atkins R, *Dr. Atkins' Vita-Nutrient Solution: Nature's Answer to Drugs,* New York: Simon & Schuster, 1998:211–215.

Boucher BJ, "Inadequate vitamin D status: Does it contribute to the disorders comprising syndrome 'X'?" *British Journal of Nutrition,* 1998;79:315–327.

Facchini F, Coulston AM, Reaven GM, "Relation between dietary vitamin intake and resistance to insulin-mediated glucose disposal in healthy volunteers," *American Journal of Clinical Nutrition,* 1996;63:946–949.

Horrobin DF, *Treatment of Diabetic Neuropathy: A New Approach,* Edinburgh: Churchill Livingstone, 1992.

Middleton E, Anne S, "Quercetin inhibits lipopolysaccharide-induced expression of endothelial cell tracellular adhesion molecule-1," *International Archives of Allergy and Immunology,* 1995;107:435–436.

Singh RB, Niaz MA, Rastogi SS, et al., "Effect of hydrosoluble coenzyme Q_{10} on blood pressure and insulin resistance in hypertensive patients with coronary artery disease," *Journal of Human Hypertension,* 1999;13:203–208.

Chapter 16. Herbal Remedies for Syndrome X

Ali M, Thomson M, "Consumption of a garlic clove a day could be beneficial in preventing thrombosis," *Prostaglandins, Leukotrines, Essential Fatty Acids,* 1995;53:211–212.

Baskaran K, "Antidiabetic effect of a leaf extract from *Gymnema sylvestre* in non-insulin-dependent diabetes mellitus patients," *Journal of Ethnopharmacology,* 1990;30:295–305.

Bordia A, Verma SK, Srivastava KC, "Effect of ginger (*Zingiber officinale Rosc*) and fenugreek (*Trigonella foenumgraecum L.*) on blood lipids, blood sugar and platelet aggregation in patients with coronary artery disease," *Prostaglandins, Leukotrines, and Essential Fatty Acids,* 1997;56:379–384.

Curi R, Alvarez M, Bazoote RB, et al., "Effect of *Stevia rebaudiana* on glucose tolerance in normal adult subjects," *Brazilian Journal of Medicine and Biological Research,* 1986;19:771–774.

Jain AK, et al., "Can garlic reduce levels of serum lipids? A controlled clinical study," *American Journal of Medicine,* 1993;94:632–635.

Kiesewetter H, et al., "Effects of garlic coated tablets in peripheral arterial occlusive disease," *Clinical Investigator,* 1993;71:383–386.

Kiesewetter H, Jung F, Pindur G, "Effects of garlic on thrombocyte aggregation, microcirculation, and other risk factors," *International Journal of Clinical Pharmacology Therapeutic Toxicology,* 1991;29: 151–155.

Sarker S, Pranava M, Marita R, "Demonstration of the hypoglycemic action of *Momordica charantia* in a validated animal model of diabetes," *Pharmacological Research,* 1996;33:1–4.

Sendl A, et al., "Comparative pharmacological investigations of *Allium ursinum* and *Allium sativum*," *Planta Medica,* 1992;58:1–7.

Shanmugasundaram ERB, "Possible regeneration of the islets of Langerhans in streptozotocin-diabetic rats given *Gymnema sylvestre* leaf extracts," *Journal of Ethnopharmacology,* 1990;30:265–279.

Shanmugasundaram ERB, "Use of *Gymnema sylvestre* leaf extract in the control of blood glucose in insulin-dependent diabetes mellitus," *Journal of Ethnopharmacology,* 1990;30:281–294.

Sharma RD, Raghuram TC, Rao NS, "Effect of fenugreek seeds on blood glucose and serum lipids in type I diabetes," *European Journal of Clinical Nutrition,* 1990;44:301–306.

Singh RB, Niaz MA, Rastogi V, et al., "Hypolipidemic and antioxidant effects of fenugreek seeds and triphala as adjuncts to dietary therapy in patients with mild to moderate hypercholesterolemia," *Perfusion,* 1998;11:124–126.

Srivastava Y, et al., "Antidiabetic and adaptogenic properties of *Momordica charantia* extract: An experimental and clinical evaluation," *Phytotherapy Research,* 1993;7:285–289.

Srivastava Y, Venkatakrishna-Bhatt H, Verma Y, "Effect of *Momordica charantia Linn.* pomous acqueous extract on cataractogenesis in nurrin alloxan diabetics," *Pharmacological Research Communications,* 1988;20:201–209.

Steiner M, Khan AH, Holbert D, et al., "A double-blind crossover study in moderately hypercholesterolemic men that compared the effect of aged garlic extract and placebo administration on blood lipids," *American Journal of Clinical Nutrition,* 1996;64:866–870.

Velussi M, Cernigoi AM, Monte AD, et al., "Long-term (12 months) treatment with an anti-oxidant drug (silymarin) is effective on hyperinsulinemia, exogenous insulin need and malondialdehyde levels in cirrhotic diabetic patients," *Journal of Hepatology,* 1997;26:871–879.

Welihinda J, et al., "Effect of *Momardica charantia* on the glucose tolerance in maturity onset diabetes," *Journal of Ethnopharmacology,* 1986;17:277–282.

Wenzel S, Stolte H, Soose M, "Effects of silibinin and antioxidants on high glucose-induced alterations of fibronectin turnover in human mesangial cell cultures," *Journal of Pharmacology and Experimental Therapeutics,* 1996;279:1520–1526.

Zeyuan D, Bingyin T, Xiaolin L, "Effect of green tea and black tea on the blood glucose, the blood triglyceride, and antioxidation in aged rats," *Journal of Agricultural and Food Chemistry,* 1998;46: 3875–3878.

INDEX